SY

5:2
YOUR
LIFE

Emma Cook is an editor for the *Guardian* and a writer specialising in parenting, psychology and relationships. ecent convert to the 5:2 diet, she decided to adapt its inciples to other areas of her life and saw fantastic its. She is also the author of the parenting advice boo *Ask Your Father – How to Answer Awkward Questions en Ask*. She lives in London with her husband and u children.

D0227373

5:2

YOUR
LIFE

**How the revolutionary
5:2 approach can transform your
HEALTH, WEALTH and HAPPINESS**

613. 25

Emma Cook

HUTCHINSON

Published by Hutchinson 2014

3 5 7 9 10 8 6 4 2

Copyright © Emma Cook 2014

Emma Cook has asserted her right under the Copyright, Designs and Patents Act, 1988, to be identified as the author of this work

This book is sold subject to the condition that it shall not, by way of trade or otherwise, be lent, resold, hired out, or otherwise circulated without the publisher's prior consent in any form of binding or cover other than that in which it is published and without a similar condition, including this condition, being imposed on the subsequent purchaser.

First published in Great Britain in 2014 by Hutchinson
Random House,
20 Vauxhall Bridge Road,
London SW1V 2SA

www.randomhouse.co.uk

Addresses for companies within The Random House Group Limited can be found at: www.randomhouse.co.uk/offices.htm

The Random House Group Limited Reg. No. 954009

A CIP catalogue record for this book is available from the British Library

ISBN 9780091954345

The publishers and author wish to thank the experts and specialists on page 268 and the following for their kind permission to reproduce extracts of their work: Oliver Burkeman; Elizabeth Day; Tim Dowling; Beeban Kidron; and Zoe Williams.

Mocktail recipes reproduced courtesy of Jayne Totty, www.redemptionbar.com

Extract from *The Power of Habit* by Charles Duhigg. Copyright © Charles Duhigg, 2012, used by permission of The Wylie Agency (UK) Limited.

Extracts from *The Seven Principles For Making Marriage Work* by John Gottman and Nan Silver. Copyright © John Gottman Ph.D and Nan Silver, 1999, used by permission of The Orion Publishing Group, London.

The 7-Minute Workout – instructions and related sequence of diagrams (illustrations by Ruth Murray) – reproduced with the permission of Chris Jordan of the Human Performance Institute, a division of Wellness & Prevention, Inc.

The Random House Group Limited supports the Forest Stewardship Council® (FSC®), the leading international forest-certification organisation. Our books carrying the FSC label are printed on FSC®-certified paper. FSC is the only forest-certification scheme supported by the leading environmental organisations, including Greenpeace. Our paper procurement policy can be found at www.randomhouse.co.uk/environment

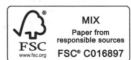

Typeset by carrdesignstudio.com

Printed and bound in Great Britain by CPI group(UK) Ltd, Croydon, CR0 4YY

The information in this book has been compiled by way of general guidance in relation to the specific subjects addressed. It is not a substitute and not to be relied on for medical, healthcare, pharmaceutical or other professional advice on specific circumstances and in specific locations. Please consult your GP before changing, stopping or starting any medical treatment. So far as the author is aware the information given is correct and up to date as at November 2013. Practice, laws and regulations all change, and the reader should obtain up to date professional advice on any such issues. The author and publishers disclaim, as far as the law allows, any liability arising directly or indirectly from the use, or misuse, of the information contained in this book

CONTENTS

5:2 Your Life   7

1.   5:2 Your Drink   27
2.   5:2 Your Fitness   59
3.   5:2 Your Finance   91
4.   5:2 Your Productivity   123
5.   5:2 Your Screen Life   153
6.   5:2 Your Relationship   179
7.   5:2 Your Worry   209
8.   5:2 Your Environment   235

Acknowledgements   267
Selected Bibliography   269
Selected Further Reading   277
Index   278

5:2

YOUR LIFE

We know that the 5:2 diet has been a phenomenal success – many thousands of us have tried it at some point over the last year. Dieters evangelise as much about the principle of 5:2 as the effects. Everyone instantly understands its premise: that this isn't about deprivation, but about enjoying whatever you want – just not all of the time. It's a technique that doesn't overtax your willpower; if it's demanding, it is also very temporary.

Elemental to its philosophy is the fact that self-denial seven days a week is not only joyless but pointless: one consistent finding among 5:2 dieters is that they have more success committing to two strict days than restricting themselves everyday.

So enjoying your freedom when you can – five days a week – means you're more likely to keep the weight off. Treating yourself to that slice of cheesecake or a plate of chips isn't a sign of weakness but intrinsic to success. This approach relies on the truism that what is permanently forbidden is inevitably much more desirable and irresistible. But, once you're allowed whatever you fancy tomorrow – just not today – it loses its allure. What a crucial difference that makes, and could make to every aspect of your life.

No-one is saying that fasting twice a week isn't a commitment. Resisting temptation for less than half the week can still feel tough. The 5:2 formula does demand will and discipline, for a short time. Which is why it is satisfying when you achieve it; small mini-hurdles that boost your motivation without dominating or reducing the rest of your life in any way.

THE SPREAD OF 5:2

Such a powerful premise was bound to transcend simply eating and, before long, it had caught the public imagination. One Sunday paper commentator noted, 'The latest trend is for the 5:2 diet … But what if our problem is information overload rather than binge-eating? And what if we cut out email instead of food groups, abstaining from perpetual connectedness for just two days a week? It might make us all a little bit saner. At least it will give me more time to start yoga, plant vegetables and learn Spanish.'

Magazines couldn't help giving it a more populist spin. There was talk in one that Jennifer Aniston was in a 5:2 relationship, only seeing her boyfriend at weekends because 'when they do see each other, they appreciate each other so much more'. Another writer expanded on the joys of being a 5:2 socialist, living by your principles without compromising your lifestyle i.e. sending your kids to state school while sipping Prosecco. So 5:2 rapidly became a byword and currency for any lifestyle or set of beliefs that could be enjoyed part-time and in moderation.

Beyond the parody, however, was also the implication that this was very much a ratio for our times, a flexible solution to the often overwhelming demands of modern living. We all want to feel we can control the temptations and prizes that come with these demands – food, alcohol, money and technology in particular. However, no one wants to give them up completely. So here was a blueprint for modern living that promised the best of both worlds, a chance to break off from these habits to exercise moderation and restraint, without the pain of total abstinence. That's when I began to think about how I could apply the 5:2 approach to the rest of my life too.

MY FIRST EXPERIENCE WITH 5:2

I had tried out different diets at various times of my life, always ending up in the same cycle of failure that can be summed up as follows: lose weight, lose willpower; comfort eat to compensate for a sense of failure; gain all lost weight, and probably a bit more too. Pick another diet, start said cycle all over again.

For the last fifteen years, I had been happy with my weight, until I became pregnant a third time in my mid-forties. For the first time, my post-birth body refused to snap back and parts of me were beginning to resemble a melted candle; I wasn't eating or drinking any more than I used to but somehow the pounds went on.

Around that time, it was difficult to ignore the many 5:2 books out there. I had never bought a diet book in my life but this time, along with many others, I tried it. Within weeks I was a convert, as much to the philosophy behind it as the results, which were impressive too. By last summer, I had dropped 13 pounds in four months and have kept it off with simple maintenance: fasting one day each week – 6:1 – aided, of course, by my 5:2 Fitness Plan.

Along with the physical benefits, I discovered some psychological ones too. I began to appreciate flavours more, savour my wine rather than gulp it. I became more thoughtful about what I ate and why. Beyond the diet, my week suddenly had more contrast and contour than it used to; there were moments of real challenge and discomfort, I must admit, but then there was satisfaction that I'd got through. There would be a sense of appreciation when I woke up on a non-fast day that the day ahead was a treat because I could enjoy what I wanted again, restriction-free. Twice a week I would feel a real boost reconnecting with those positive feelings of achievement.

I also found my fast days were a time to reset and reflect, take stock of ingrained habits that I had never really challenged, until now. It certainly made me much more mindful and self-aware once I dipped back into the rhythms of my normal routine.

It happened to suit my own temperament perfectly too. Self-discipline has never been my strong point. I do have willpower but it's a limited commodity that I have to use carefully. Which is why, as a journalist, I thrive on tight deadlines, working in short, intense bursts with the promise that life may be tough for a while but, when the work has finished, I can relax and live how I please – how similar, in fact, to the 5:2 way.

A few weeks into my diet, my husband was so impressed by my uncharacteristic willpower, and the results, that he joined me – it began to work for him too and we found it even more pleasurable as a shared experience, supporting each other and comparing notes.

We agreed it felt strangely satisfying and inspiring to step outside our normal routine, in a way that didn't feel too rigid or prescriptive, and live life differently for two days a week. Maybe because we were trying it out together, and discussed it more as a result, it felt like a significant change because it was shared.

Rather than both slumping in front of the telly twice a week, in a languid, weary blur from the usual combination of pasta and wine, we were more alert and lively.

We stayed up later, talked and made plans, finished unread books. My husband enthused that he slept better and felt far more refreshed on his post-5:2-day mornings. Both of us looked forward to treating ourselves that evening too, knowing that we could indulge in a nice meal together.

Along with our diet, our shopping habits inevitably altered. We had to work harder to make our fast meals more satisfying, with fresher, more unusual ingredients, which meant fewer convenience foods from supermarkets. My husband ordered a weekly local veg box so he could cook ahead for our 5:2 days, and there was enough left over – black carrot soup anyone? – to take into work for lunch too. Soon we were totting up how much money we were saving, not only on food and alcohol twice a week, but also the creeping costs of sandwiches at work.

As we began to combine these changes with more exercise, to maintain the effects of the diet, we both began to realise that one small change was a catalyst for so many others. Eating and drinking, the way we enjoyed our leisure time and became more conscious of saving money – this felt like a more holistic approach than a simple diet plan.

I wondered if this powerful premise was too good to restrict to weight loss and that it was more than possible to broaden the potential of the 5:2 tool kit: why couldn't the ratio of restriction versus freedom work in every context where we want to challenge and refine our habits and routines?

Why not introduce it to my family too, I thought, as I saw my three children – 11, 10 and 2 years old – hooked to their various electronic devices. I knew it would be unrealistic to deny them these screens altogether, and it never seemed to work when we tried rationing them to certain hours during the day; hitting that perfect balance was often a subject that

11

came up with other parents I spoke to.

Already I had slowly begun to feel more uncomfortable about the effects of internet use – in our own lives as well as our children's. In her recent documentary *InRealLife*, filmmaker Beeban Kidron focuses on teenagers and their relationship with their screens and smartphones. She wrote about her film, commenting that 'asking a young person to put down their Xbox, shut their computer or stop looking at their smartphone is like asking an alcoholic to put down their drink.' She also notes the relationship between a parent's screen life and their children. 'What surprised me was the anger of many teenagers who, in turn, felt abandoned by parents whose own eyes were fixed on electronic devices.'

I admit that my own relationship with my laptop and iPhone certainly wasn't helping matters. So after my success with the diet, and knowing how my willpower benefited from short durations of abstinence, I knew it was a good opportunity to 5:2 my screen life, as well as my children's – you can read all about the results in 5:2 Your Screen Life.

Although there were challenges, it was – and still is – a realistic routine that works for all of us. So Mondays and Thursdays remain screen-free in our household – two weekday evenings that are a lot noisier and more argumentative, but also less passive and self-absorbed too. The children interact more, read to the youngest, help me out in the kitchen; I could never go back to the way we were.

Once we established our screen diet, the infinite possibilities that 5:2 could shape felt exciting to me. I was enthusing to my editor at *Guardian Weekend* magazine about my new 'multi-5:2' approach. Within weeks, the magazine had devoted a whole issue to it where writers, including myself, had to 5:2 different aspects of their lives for a month, and we were all genuinely surprised by the benefits.

At this point, it was only really my family that had benefited from the 5:2 approach, but now the concept had gone public and, judging by the huge response to the feature, I felt it had much wider potential.

A CULTURE OF CRAVING

Fasting has been with us for thousands of years – the notion that abstinence can purify the mind and benefit the body has enduring appeal. Early followers included Ancient Greek philosophers Plato and Hippocrates, while many religions, including Buddhism, Islam and Christianity, require fasting as an act of penance and faith, to cleanse the soul as well as increase endurance and test willpower.

In a way, the idea of abstaining twice a week, to withdraw, focus and increase self-discipline, is a very twenty-first-century antidote to our current eating habits. As a nation, we are increasingly eating to excess, in particular refined carbohydrates. Anyone who has children will know it's a continual battle to escape the presence of fast-food, snacks and fizzy drinks, and to stick to three sensible meals a day. This culture of constant availability is, inevitably, impacting on our health. According to NHS figures, there has been a marked increase in obesity rates over the past eight years. In 1993, 13 per cent of men and 16 per cent of women were obese – in 2011 this rose to 24 per cent for men and 26 per cent for women. For children starting at primary school in 2011, 9.5 per cent were obese.

Partly the 5:2 diet is a response to these ever more extreme trends. Yet we know that other areas of our life follow a similar pattern, where we continually graze on all manner of modern pastimes, with increasingly less time off in between. Twitter, Instagram, Facebook, texts, emails, games, shopping, telly – all these are technology's 'refined carbohydrates', and they're equally addictive. These activities dominate our time, with boundaries between work and leisure, weekdays and weekends becoming ever more indistinct. Just like the blurring between snacking and mealtimes. We've somehow unlearnt the ability to exist in a contented state of not consuming.

We never really hunger for anything any more, but we do crave. We crave another 'hit', diversion and form of escapism – the next snack, drink, dress, DVD, online game, tweet or text. We anticipate and yearn for these, even though – when they come – they never really satisfy us. This perpetual state of restless consumer 'snacking' on everything, including food, has huge commercial advantage, which is why it's encouraged, but it doesn't appear to make us any happier.

THE BIRTH OF 5:2

In the beginning, there was 5:2, or in fact 6:1, according to Exodus: 'Six days a week you shall work, but on the seventh day you shall rest.' God also abided by the 6:1 ratio – efficiently creating the heavens and earth in six days. Up until the 1800s, a six-day work week was standard, and the term 'weekend' didn't slip into common currency until 1878.

The two-day break only really became a permanent fixture when car manufacturer Henry Ford discovered, after years of research, that 5:2 was the perfect quotient for maximum productivity – you'll discover how to put it to good use in 5:2 Your Productivity. He ran a number of experiments, concluding that forty hours a week over five days is the optimum output. Any more hours – or days – than that and the standard starts to decline. Another benefit in giving his workers Saturday off was, he hoped, to encourage them to spend their hard-earned wages and drive more.

The weekend was also a natural full stop, the only time that you could shop in a frantic working week; also a time to rest, go to church, reflect and withdraw. Gradually, though, as the twenty-first century has progressed, the weekend has become something of an endangered species.

Arguably, it was only a matter of time before a new variation on 5:2 would come into being, possibly not one that Ford would have recognised, but a twenty-first-century version that offers a similar space for rest and reflection, as well as a helpful ratio to boost motivation and productivity.

WHY THESE EIGHT AREAS?

In *5:2 Your Life*, I wanted to include eight chapters that touch on key aspects of modern life. Some involve the habits we indulge in and enjoy, possibly to our detriment, and that we know require moderation – spending money, drinking and using technology more than fulfil this remit.

Then there are those habits that would benefit our lives, and those around us, if they were increased not reduced, that are elemental to individual and collective wellbeing in different ways: these are fitness, productivity and environment.

Finally, I chose two emotional elements – relationships and worry – that are the potential victims, if you like, of our more compulsive habits, which is why I devote a chapter to each. I felt that all the areas had to pass a basic rule: that they are healthy enough to enjoy in moderation and don't demand total abstinence – which is why you won't find 5:2 Your Smoking in my chapters.

Each one is here because it connects and informs the other, increases our self-awareness, and allows us to examine our own personalities and what truly motivates us.

5:2 YOUR LIFE – THE PHILOSOPHY

You may well be reading this because you're a fan of the 5:2 diet and hope that such a simple premise can work as well across the rest of your life too. I can assure you that it will. As with the diet, the *5:2 Your Life* philosophy isn't extreme. You choose the area of your life you'd like to change, turn to that chapter, and try to focus on that area for just two days each week with the help of the seven-step plan you'll find there. Some days, and weeks, will be better than others. You can move slowly, step-by-step, as I did when I first attempted to 5:2 my children's screen life. In the first week or two, I felt I was meeting constant resistance from my children and occasionally I even weakened and went 6:1, letting them on their screens for short bursts. I didn't feel this was evidence to give up. I simply encouraged them to start where we left off on our next 5:2 day. Overall we were always moving in the right direction until, after a month or two, we didn't even realise we were doing it any more, and the two-day screen break became an unconscious family habit.

The same is true for every other area of *5:2 Your Life*. If you aim for perfection seven days a week, you're inviting failure. Instead, you can move at a pace that suits you, whether it's going offline, spending less money, cutting your alcohol units, working more productively, exercising more or helping the environment.

What unifies each chapter is my own experience: from Screen to Finance, Drink to Fitness, Relationship to Productivity and Worry to Environment, each area has touched on a personal story that I felt was crucial to shaping the advice and techniques offered in the steps.

Key to this is the idea of how creative and productive a temporary constraint can be – when we can't do a certain thing and we have to try something new, the results can be unexpected.

For example, if you walk to work for one day a week, rather than drive, you will almost certainly become healthier, and save money too, and you can feel satisfied that you're cutting your carbon footprint. But there are other benefits to walking that you can't guess at until you try a new variation. It could be noticing your environment more, looking up at buildings, chatting to new neighbours.

There are incidental gains to be made every time you decide to take a different route, choose a different meal or a different seat, omit one habit and introduce another. Part of the 5:2 philosophy is to challenge routines and be more spontaneous, knowing that if you behave in the same way that you always have done, seven days a week, nothing will ever change.

Constraints can offer something else too – a fixed time to achieve a goal; in other words, a deadline. We all lack willpower to some extent; it's a precious commodity that should be used sparingly within a short time frame.

As productivity expert Tony Schwarz says, 'We all work best in intervals, we're better in waves rather than linear output – short bursts.' This is a principle that applies as much to productivity as fitness, as you'll read in the relevant chapters. You can view 5:2 as the ultimate interval workout, ring-fencing two days a week to stretch yourself in whatever area you choose, with the comfort of knowing that tomorrow is already in sight.

'When something is open-ended, no defined period of time … you won't be fully engaged. Why can a sprinter run at the highest possible speed for an entire race? Because there's a visible ending. You can handle anything when you know you'll be stopping soon,' adds Schwarz.

Also key to the 5:2 approach is the importance of replacing instant gratification with long-term rewards. This means genuine examination and reflection on why certain habits are so appealing, what triggers them, and why you enjoy the payoff. Only then is long-lasting change sustainable.

Author Charles Duhigg writes in his comprehensive study, *The Power of Habit*, 'Researchers ... discovered a simple neurological loop at the core of every habit, a loop that consists of three parts: a cue, a routine, and a reward ... Once you have diagnosed the habit loop of a particular behavior, you can look for ways to supplant old vices with new routines.'

The best place to start is to simply stop – be it opening the fridge for a snack when you're not really hungry, switching on the TV when you don't really want to watch it, buying something online that you're not sure you really want, checking for emails repeatedly. All these are reflexive habits that you probably don't even question, and it's only when you ask yourself 'How would I feel if I stopped doing that?' that you can understand what you're trying to avoid and escape.

Professor Mark Williams, co-author of *Mindfulness: A Practical Guide to Finding Peace in a Frantic World* with Dr Danny Penman, explains, 'What you'll notice with 5:2 is how powerful your habits are and you'll only see it when you try to stop it. It's like going against the tide or a current which is automatic habit. It can feel quite painful: you never realised that this habit was so compelling.'

In my case, on my 5:2 diet days and my alcohol-free evenings, what popped up as I was pushing against the riptide of ingrained habits was simple boredom. My trigger to reach inside the fridge, graze between meals, top up my wine glass, surf shopping websites, all sprang from this emotion. Once I was able to notice this in a suitably mindful and detached way, thanks to the mindfulness meditation exercises in 5:2 Your Worry, I knew I needed to create alternative rewards. So delicious juices rather than wine on my alcohol-free nights, spending virtually nothing twice a week with the promise I can go for a nice meal once a month, and making sure I update my iPod playlist so I've got an incentive to exercise; all these tricks help to maintain my new habits.

Concentrating on one area of your life two days a week feels long enough to experience the possibilities of change, and to feel that potential permeate the rest of the week.

On those other five days, you'll be free. If you want you can indulge online, drink more wine, eat meat, forget about exercise, impulse-buy, drive your car and to hell with your carbon footprint. In reality, it may not work like this, hopefully because you'll want to combine lots of *5:2 Your Life* areas, which will make you generally more thoughtful and moderate overall, and keener not to undo all that good work once you feel the benefits.

We know there must be a better, healthier balance, physically and emotionally. I believe the 5:2 ratio can help put us back in touch with every aspect of our lives.

THE BENEFITS OF COMBINING

Until I began developing *5:2 Your Life*, I had never followed a self-help guide. Even though – perhaps because – I have written for twenty years about personality, behaviour and relationships, I was the least likely person to be convinced by a simple premise or plan that could change things dramatically.

I really wasn't sure what the results would be when I went on a mission to apply the 5:2 formula to every aspect of my life.

The benefit to my screen life had been significant enough but, as I experimented with different areas, combining one or two here, experimenting with another there, I began to realise there was a cumulative effect. What I learnt in one area would inform another – for instance, when I tried a high-intensity workout technique in my running routine, I knew it could help with my productivity, working in intense timed bursts.

Planning our meals and cooking in batches made me think more about saving money, which in turn led me to be more receptive to the benefits in 5:2 Your Environment, consuming less or only eating meat twice a week.

Surprising connections, comparisons, personal insights and payoffs began to pop up everywhere once I started to combine lots of different areas of my life. A certain truth or 'bigger picture' begins to emerge about your personality; how your values and beliefs in one area shape and define your behaviour in another. In isolation, simply focusing on, say, diet, alcohol or fitness, I'm convinced the journey and the experience wouldn't have been so rewarding. Nor would I have learnt so much about myself.

MAKING IT WORK FOR YOU

When I first started on a mission to 5:2 every area of my life, I wasn't sure what to expect or how encouraging the experts I encountered along the way would be – would their research and experience support my idea?

The answer has been a unanimous yes. Without exception, the many specialists I have talked to at length – in psychology and psychotherapy, fitness, culture, productivity, environment, finance, drink, technology, relationships and worry – have all embraced this ratio, instantly grasping how it can impact our lives.

Whatever their area of research and expertise, the same message comes through: consistently altering our behaviour for a fraction of each week creates all sorts of unique and unexpected benefits for all the week, for good.

The input and advice from these experts for every life area is crucial and invaluable; their wisdom shapes and defines each section.

When I was developing the 5:2 life plan, I thought a great deal about what each chapter could offer in terms of ultimate achievement and accomplishment. In the 5:2 diet, weight loss is a quantifiable goal, but how would you measure, say, relationships or environment? Would it be more intangible? Not necessarily. I was determined that in each life area there should be clear and measurable results. So in 5:2 Your Environment, I only recommend habit changes that, for two days a week, will measurably reduce your carbon footprint and create other payoffs across your other life areas that you can enjoy from Day 1. I call these 5:2 full houses – where one new habit will help you gain in at least one other life area, i.e. using your car less and cycling will earn you green points but will also save you money (5:2 Your Finance) and make you healthier (5:2 Your Fitness), increasing your wellbeing and reducing stress (5:2 Your Worry).

5:2 Your Life is a one-stop shop to making lasting change, and the following chapters will show you how. With no complicated rules, each chapter offers a clear and flexible strategy through a seven-step plan that weaves in my own experience alongside advice and testimonies from the many people who have already found how well it works for them and were keen to report back exactly how.

Some of the steps are written exercises that you can complete on one of your two 5:2 days and other steps offer practical techniques and advice on alternative activities for your 5:2 days. Since the life areas are so diverse, so then is the advice – you'll find a section on 5:2 mocktails to make your non-alcohol days a pleasure not a deprivation; detailed diagrams to help you through 5:2 fitness workouts; music playlists to run to; and exercises to 5:2 your sex life.

Almost every 5:2 life area begins with an audit, allowing you to step back and examine your habits – be it how much you spend, drink, worry or exercise. Often you'll be encouraged to keep a diary, record your usage before and after you embark on your 5:2 life plan, using it as a benchmark to return to, charting your progress and reassessing your goals and motivations. These goals and motivations are essential, so you know how to measure your success and can be clear about your incentives when the two days get tough.

HOW LONG SHOULD I DO IT ALL FOR?

Since the *5:2 Your Life* approach is so broad, I'm not offering a twenty-one-day programme for every habit you would like to improve, whether it's helping the planet, worrying less or being more productive. Yes, you'll be able to measure results as soon as you start, across all chapters, but this isn't a finite approach to change. It's up to you how long you spend on each life area – you may dip in and out of different ones, returning at a later date to refresh and update your progress.

What this plan will do is help you live life in a more satisfying way, where you won't feel deprived but rewarded instead. Just like the diet, you'll find 5:2 Your Life realistic and easy to maintain, informing your daily life but certainly not dominating it.

IT'S FINE TO FAIL

5:2 Your Life works on the assumption that we lead busy lives with habits that we're pretty attached to, so dramatic changes to our routines that demand perfection are not going to work. On this plan, we can have moments of weakness when we won't want to stick to a plan. As I've said, rather like the 5:2 diet, it may be a moderate approach, but that doesn't mean it won't sometimes be testing. If it isn't, then you're probably not doing it right.

The beauty of 5:2, as we've established, indulging in a little of what you want is built into the formula. So you feel a bit under the weather and you can't face your high-intensity fitness routine, who cares? A couple of days later, energy levels restored, you will be happy to knuckle down to that brief workout. The odd deviation or slip is fine; just pick up where you left off. View it as a long, slow burn, if you like. Being kind to yourself, and acknowledging the odd diversion won't make any sort of permanent dent in your overall dedication.

WHICH AREAS AND WHICH DAYS?

As I discovered after my initial 5:2 foray with my family, alter one link in the chain, and many other parts are affected too. Like painting one wall of your house white, you'll find it will throw the other three into sharp relief. So my 5:2 diet shone a light on many other aspects of my life.

When I applied 5:2 across the spectrum, I began with diet, which I haven't included in my book because I feel it's extensively covered elsewhere. Nevertheless, it's an easy win if you're eating less twice a week to avoid alcohol too. I chose different days to 5:2 my screen life and diet because I realised, initially, that I needed a full stomach to negotiate with grumpy children who have been denied their devices.

Another payoff from my diet was saving money, which I developed further in 5:2 Your Finance and which I soon discovered was a natural complement to 5:2 Your Environment I was already running at least twice a week, but as I researched the ultimate 5:2 Fitness Plan, I applied the interval protocol to my runs and was able to cut back on my exercise by a couple of days.

That freed up a little more time to focus on worry, which combined well with my fitness, as well as my productivity. Relationships slipped in neatly with offscreen days, spending more time talking or enjoying a night out.

So you can see from the table opposite how possible it is to combine all eight areas and still enjoy Saturday off!

It may sound daunting tackling a few chapters simultaneously, but it is surprisingly achievable and enjoyable too. However, you certainly don't have to try all of them at the same time. You can also use the table as a guide to where your 5:2 days for just one or two different life areas could fall. For instance, ideally your alcohol-free days should come after one another to give your system maximum time to rejuvenate. Monday also feels like the right time to abstain from various indulgences after the weekend, which is why several are highlighted here, but this certainly isn't set in stone. The appeal of *5:2 Your Life* is its flexibility: you can embark on one chapter and combine with another or simply work through them in order. Once you've tried the exercises and techniques in some areas, say the relationship chapter, you'll find that it's more a case of being mindful about what you've already learnt, aware of one or two key insights or techniques that will apply to other chapters too. *5:2 Your Life* is a discreet way of making a big difference, without intrusive or complicated rules and changes.

	Monday	Tuesday	Wednesday	Thursday	Friday	Saturday	Sunday
Free						✓	
Drink	✓	✓					
Environment	✓		✓				
Productivity	✓			✓			
Relationship	✓				✓		
Screen	✓			✓			
Finance	✓		✓				
Worry		✓		✓			
Fitness			✓				✓

For example, if you're using the meditation exercises from 5:2 Your Worry twice a week, these should take no longer than fifteen or twenty minutes and can be combined with your warm-down from the 5:2 Fitness Plan, which shouldn't take more than twenty minutes either – that's less than an hour to commit to two different 5:2 life areas.

Once you get the hang of one area and feel the benefits, you'll naturally make links with other ones too, creating different patterns that suit your own lifestyle.

By now I hope you can see the potential of this holistic approach as well as the insights and tools you can expect from each chapter. What's important is to feel excited about trying it out, changing your outlook to make you feel more energetic and alive, healthier, wealthier and happier. That's the simple promise of *5:2 Your Life*.

5:2

YOUR DRINK

LIFE BEFORE MY 5:2 DRINK DIET

Wednesday evening and I've crossed the finishing line of the nightly marathon that is the children's bedtime. 'Wine o'clock!' a gleeful inner voice announces as I almost skip down the stairs into the kitchen where my husband is cooking our meal. Toys have been pushed to the margins, lights are low, serenity restored and, most importantly, he's pouring something chilled and white into two glasses. Ah, that sound as the golden liquid swirls around my glass. No other ritual is so pleasing, so untarnished by frequent repetition and routine.

When I first met my husband, he managed a wine shop, so you could say wine has been a shared interest, right there at the start of our relationship, and it still is a shared means of enjoying the end of the day. As we've grown older, more aware of eating healthily and exercising, alcohol is the only aspect of our diet that has somehow escaped our scrutiny, probably because we can't quite bear to let it go. It signifies a time when we could be spontaneous, go out at a moment's notice, be more carefree. It still makes us feel like partners in crime, our covert secret. 'Shall I … you know,' he raises an eyebrow when we realise there's nothing in the fridge, 'pop to the shop for "provisions"?' he asks, as the children go to bed.

But as time goes on, I wonder how it looks from my children's perspective. They see us drinking wine at weekends (we manage to wait until they're in bed during the week). Every so often, my 11- and 10-year-old will ask for a sip and we'll say, 'No – something to try when you're older.' That 'something', they know, is associated with winding down, relaxing and pleasure. Will that knowledge shape their own habits, influence how much they drink each week?

How does this make me feel? Certainly not guilty enough to abstain every night but, like the rest of my friends, I feel a mix of unease and anxiety with the current situation. One friend recently confessed that she has her first glass of wine at half five when she cooks her 4-year-old's tea, to help her destress. 'Is it bad he notices?' she asks.

Along with the guilt, there is a sense that we are part of a new generation of parents. Our parents never used to drink like this. When I grew up, a bottle of wine at Sunday lunch was a rare treat. Yet for my generation, who married and had children later, drinking was part of our young adult lives, something we'd think about giving up at some point, but not quite yet. Until recently, that is. Maybe it's middle age, along with a nagging sense of unease as the children grow more aware and knowing, but I knew that I wanted to drink less, and hopefully feel more energetic and healthy as a result.

Of course worrying about drinking each night isn't the preserve of weary parents.

We don't even have that excuse of feeling like we deserve a reward, because we don't have children, but we still enjoy that nightly ritual. My boyfriend and I come home from work, share the cooking while we listen to music, chat about the day and, without fail, open a bottle of wine. By the time we get to the meal, we're often over halfway through and we'll have a glass from the next one while we settle down to watch a box set. I worry that I actually reassure myself by saying, "Well, we only had the one glass each from a second bottle" – as if that's restrained!

Andrea, 30

In the past, I've found it easy to give up alcohol in January and have gone on to cut down for a few weeks after that, but then, like so many people, I would lapse. I'd be back to having wine most weekday evenings. Instead, I needed a new weekly routine I could stick to, where permanent moderation, not abstinence, was the ideal.

Reassuringly, abstinence may not be desirable anyway. A paper that came out three years ago in the journal *Alcoholism: Clinical and Experimental Research* suggests that abstainers' (people who are not current drinkers) mortality rates are higher than those of heavy drinkers. The researchers, at the University of Texas, looked at mortality rates over twenty years, and discovered that they were lowest among moderate drinkers – defined in the study as one to three drinks a day.

Abstaining may not be that helpful in terms of teaching children how to drink sensibly either. Instead, drinking moderately in front of them, where they can see alcohol isn't relied upon, should be viewed as a social responsibility, an essential parenting skill rather than a guilty pleasure, something I'm happy to drink to on my 5:2 Drink Diet.

The wind-down wine at home is only half the picture. Social drinking can be at least as harmful and habit-forming. Paula, 36, works in the City, and her pattern of consumption was the opposite to that of the weary at-home parent. She used to abstain through the week and drink heavily all weekend, arriving at the office most Monday mornings acutely hungover. 'It was a way of controlling my drinking because I knew once I had one wine, I'd drink the whole bottle. I was very all or nothing.' Paula wanted to master moderate drinking, rather than feeling so polarised, by trusting herself more during the week and building self-confidence so that she could pace herself without drinking too much in one go.

MAKING THE 5:2 CONNECTION

When I began the 5:2 diet, fasting twice a week, I knew I had to cut out drinking too. I wondered how difficult this would be – that evening ritual was as ingrained as flossing each morning and switching on the radio. But once I realised that my two glasses were around 250 calories in total – half my fast-day allowance, it felt like a no-brainer. I was also relieved to find out I didn't rely on that drink at the end of the day as much as I thought – it was a big psychological boost to know I could get rid of a habit that had hung around me for so long. Saving money and feeling better the next day was an added perk.

And something else interesting happened on my 5:2 diet day. By 7 p.m. each evening, uppermost in my mind was food, not drink. How promiscuous and easily distracted my brain could be, I realised.

The 5:2 diet doesn't last for ever, or even that long – the reason being that it actually works – so within a few months I found

I only needed to maintain my desired weight with one weekly fast. However, I still wanted to stick to two or three alcohol-free days (AFDs) each week but, off the 5:2 diet, I knew I'd have to find other ways to divert myself from reaching for a glass.

I approached Dr James Nicholls, research manager for Alcohol Research UK, who was enthusiastic about the 5:2 ratio, and how suitable it would be for a certain type of drinker. 'The 24–44-year-olds have the highest consumption in the country. The 5:2 approach has a resonance and simplicity to it and would speak well to this cohort of drinkers, many of whom are in the habit of drinking at home. It's something people can make sense of, so they can break a routine which creates a window for behavioural change.'

Andrew Langford, chief executive at the British Liver Trust, can also see the gains. 'One of our main mantras is that people need at least two consecutive days off, and so this is a great message to adopt. It's good to rest your whole system and to allow your liver this time to rejuvenate.'

THE 5:2 DRINK DIET; aims and benefits

- It's a simple approach that will change your attitude to alcohol, from a practical as well as a psychological perspective.

- The easy-to-follow and pragmatic rules will guarantee you stick to at least two AFDs a week and cut units overall.

- You will feel happier, sleep better and have more energy.

- Your self-confidence will increase as you realise you can control when and what you drink, and that you are able to forget alcohol easily on your AFDs.

- You can still enjoy alcohol for much of the time but you will appreciate it in a new and different way.

- Tapping into the positive feeling you enjoy the morning after your AFDs each week will strengthen your motivation and fire up the incentive to carry on.

- You will realise the potential health benefits of cutting down: reducing your risk of raised blood pressure, liver damage and many types of cancer.

- You will enjoy new activities and experiences, viewing your AFDs as opportunities to do something different, rather than as joyless drink-free days to endure.

GETTING STARTED ON THE 5:2 DRINK DIET

Now you've read about my experience, and heard about some of the risks of social drinking, here's how you put the 5:2 Drink Diet into practice. These seven steps will offer a unique combination of practical tips, journal exercises and self-reflection to help you through your AFDs – and your drink days too.

Work through the steps on your AFDs, starting with a drink audit and journal. Steps 4–7 should be viewed as works-in-progress that you can return to as often as you want.

SEVEN STEPS TO MAKE THE 5:2 DRINK DIET WORK FOR YOU

1

Do a drink audit

Whether you're a social drinker who wants to cut down, or a mother who looks forward to her 'little helper' once the children are in bed, now is the time to confront one simple truth. How much do you really drink? Being honest – with yourself, never mind with anyone else – can be more challenging than you think. When researchers at University College London compared alcohol sales figures with surveys of what people claimed they drank, there was a significant discrepancy. They were far in excess of official figures, with 19 per cent more men than previously thought drinking in excess of the recommended daily limit, and 26 per cent more women. Weekly consumption was much higher than people admitted, too, with 15 per cent more men and 11 per cent more women drinking above weekly guideline limits.

So be warned, and remember, the more realistic you are now, the more chance these steps will help kick-start your 5:2 drink routine. Donna Cornett, psychologist and founder of Drink Link Moderation, says, 'You can't underestimate the value of monitoring – research shows that if you count the number of drinks you have daily, you'll automatically cut down on them because of that simple awareness.'

Sit down and, as accurately as you are able, list what you've consumed over the last week. This isn't so easy in retrospect, so be patient with yourself. Aim for three columns: list drinks down one side, units in the middle (see Drink Facts, pp.56–8, for the number of units in your favourite alcoholic drink) and, for shock value, calories in the final margin. Now, add these up to give yourself a snapshot for a day, a week and a month. Find a website that can do the drink/unit/calorie conversions for you. I found this one straightforward and helpful: www.drinkaware.co.uk /understand–your–drinking/unit–calculator

Over the next four weeks, as you start your 5:2 Drink Diet, keep a notebook handy to jot down your daily intake, listing amounts – number of glasses, units and, if you find it helpful, calories. These figures will be your incentive as you see the number of calories and units fall, and your Alcohol Free Days (AFDs) increase, as you follow the steps below. Within six weeks, you won't need to keep tabs because moderate drinking will be natural and automatic.

Here's how one week of my drink diary looked a few months ago.

Monday
  One medium glass of white wine – 2 units (165 calories)
Tuesday
  Two medium glasses of white wine – 4 units (330 calories)
Wednesday
  Two small glasses of white wine – 2 units (165 calories)
Thursday
  One small glass of white wine – 1 unit (82 calories)
Friday
  Two medium glasses of white wine – 4 units (330 calories)
Saturday
  Two medium glasses of white wine – 4 units (330 calories)
Sunday
  Two small glasses of white wine – 2 units (165 calories)

Total units – 19
Total calories – 1,268

' *I drink every day and have done so for years. That makes me sound like an alcoholic, but actually I just enjoy a glass of wine at the end of the day. I love the woozy feeling, how relaxed it makes me feel, the social aspect of it. At the weekends we often have meals with friends, in which case I'd drink a bottle or more on both days. I always check the alcohol content on the bottle – any lower than 13 and I feel cheated. So my alcohol audit is at least 30 units a week, sometimes 40. I am shocked it's well over the recommended amount and I know I should cut down, especially since I worry that I can feel my kidneys ache sometimes.*'

Amanda, 35

2 Set goals

Use your notes in Step 1 as a foundation for what you hope to achieve. What are your first thoughts when you examine your current intake? Are you surprised? How do your total units tally with the national guidelines? For women, these are 2–3 units per day (21 units per week) and for men 3–4 units per day (28 units per week). Bear in mind that the British Liver Trust recommends two to three *consecutive* alcohol-free days each week. Ask yourself where you would most like to improve your habits and then plan an ideal weekly intake based on your current real one. Here's how I wanted mine to look:

Monday
   5:2 fast day – AFD

Tuesday
   AFD – a consecutive day recommended by the British Liver Trust and national guidelines

Wednesday
Two smaller glasses of white wine – 3 units

Thursday
AFD

Friday
Two smaller glasses of white – 3 units

Saturday
Half-bottle of white wine – 5 units

Sunday
Two smaller glasses of white – 3 units

Total units – 14
Total calories – 1,100

So, in summary, my plan consisted of three main goals: I wanted to lower my overall units so that they would be well within weekly recommended guidelines; I intended to swap to two *consecutive* alcohol-free days to rest my liver, and I aimed to add an optional extra AFD on Thursdays. I decided to make that third alcohol-free day flexible in terms of the day on which it fell, but Monday and Tuesday are now set in stone. 'Know your drink limit and stick to it,' says Cornett. 'Instead of leaving your drinking to chance, keep those goals in the back of your mind and think about the skills and strategies you'll use to keep them in place.'

3 **Be prepared**
Changing drinking habits can be hard for some people, so begin by ensuring you are giving yourself every chance you can to succeed. Make a list of activities that inspire you and steer clear of tasks that make your spirits sink.

That means no clearing out the kitchen cupboard, ironing or filling in a tax return on your days without alcohol.

Look ahead to an evening without a drink and check your mood. Remind yourself that these two – or three – days off are a chance to do something different, enjoyable, even indulgent. How you feel as you approach your AFDs each week will determine how easily you'll slash your weekly units and make this a life change rather than a short-term resolution.

I managed to cut down drinking two to three days each week but, until recently, I viewed my AFDs as 'vanilla' days: bland and forgettable, but necessary. Sharing my AFDs with my husband certainly made it easier, but there was still an element of 'Oh well, here we go', a gloomy contrast to the usual pleasurable anticipation at suppertime. In the long term, clearly this mind-set would not have been very sustainable.

'There are other ways to think about cutting back on alcohol, looking at the positive aspects of what you can achieve,' says hypnotherapist Georgia Foster who has devised a programme aimed at moderation, called 'The Drink Less Mind'. 'Once your mind registers these changes, it's easier to do and then you'll realise you haven't had a drink for three, four or five days because you've dropped those old assumptions.'

> *I usually spend around £7 on a bottle of wine, so I have been spending that on a glossy magazine and a snack such as those treaty tapas from a posh supermarket. I still feel like I'm indulging myself, and also a bit guilty, which is the same feeling as having a drink! It gets me over the hurdle until it's not habitual to drink any more.*
> Suzanne, 29

Be aware of quick-fix diversions should a craving strike. 'Remember the first couple of hours when you get home are the most challenging,' says Foster 'Open that book you haven't read, go to that movie or a yoga class. Your brain will get used to it and connect to that new behaviour.' Make sure the fridge is well stocked with nonalcoholic mixers, juices, syrups and decent fizzy water, and don't miss out on Step 7's tasty mocktails. Reassure yourself that these nonalcoholic ingredients are still cheaper than a bottle of wine or a few beers, and they will last longer too.

> *My danger hour is making the kids' tea. It has become a habit to sit down with them with a glass of wine. So if I have something planned after the children have gone to bed, preferably something that I have to drive to, then it's a great distraction from wanting a drink. I've taken to going to aqua-aerobics with a friend – by the time I get home at 8.30 p.m., the urge to drink has faded a little. It's turned an evening of deprivation into a social event that's left me feeling super-virtuous and healthy.*
>   Jenny, 43

4 Look at your motivations

To reduce your drinking, you need to understand why you're doing it, the emotional triggers involved. Be aware of the relationship between your thoughts, feelings and actions. 'It's not about how much you even drink – it's the emotion that drives you there,' says Foster.

We're not talking necessarily about extreme situations that you can't control – losing your job, getting divorced, experiencing a bereavement – where alcohol might be an obvious escape, but the more mundane letdowns and trivial disappointments that can punctuate a day, make you feel vulnerable: a parking ticket, a poor decision at work, a truculent toddler at bedtime; all these can make you feel that the least you deserve is a drink. 'Your unconscious mind will think, "When was the last time I felt tired, let down, bored, etc. and what made me feel better?" That's when you'll instinctively crave alcohol,' says Foster.

Keeping track of what you drink is important, but getting to the root of your emotional responses is also crucial. What motivates that first drink, and then another? How do you feel when your glass is almost empty? Sit down with a pen and paper, perhaps with your partner or a friend who is willing to take part. Refer to your list in Step 1 and now sketch in the bigger picture. What frustrations in daily life make you most likely to reflexively want alcohol? Describe those times, how they make you feel – stressed, angry, anxious or otherwise.

'Really have a look at each circumstance,' advises Cornett. 'Soon you'll start to notice patterns, particularly if you overdrink at certain times. Then you can develop solutions to fix or modify your triggers.'

For me, the first drink of the day (the "bar" opens at 7 p.m. on weekdays, 6 p.m. at weekends) marks the beginning of "me" time, when I can start relaxing after work. I find the sound of the cork popping out of the wine bottle quite exhilarating: it's like a signal of freedom.

I usually cook while I drink so I find the whole experience both creative and therapeutic; I even play music too, which makes the action of drinking/cooking/listening both pleasurable and sensual. I love the woozy, cosy feeling I have after the second glass. I'm in proper relaxation mode then – ready to eat a nice meal then relax with my wife, watching a DVD or chatting.

When the bottle's finished, usually after three glasses each, I feel sated but disappointed there's no more. I want that sedated, light-headed feeling to continue but I also don't want to lose control, so would normally stop at one bottle during the week. At weekends I'll normally open another, drink half of that, then feel guilty about it the next day. And a little groggy.

I associate drinking with cosiness and relaxation. My parents drank a fair bit around me as I was growing up so I consider drinking as a sociable, deeply satisfying experience.

On days when I choose not to drink, usually twice a week, I think that my evenings will be dull and uneventful and that's where I'd like to retune my mind and see them as enjoyable in their own way.

Bill, 48

Foster also encourages her clients to be aware of the sniping inner voice that tells us we're not good enough, that we'll fail or let ourselves down. Often we turn to drink to quell these negative rumblings, she says, rather than simply dismissing them as untrue. 'If you listen to the critic inside us, believe everything it says, then you will drink more,' says Foster. We need to recognise that the same voice will say, 'Go on, you deserve a drink, you've had a tough day, so what if it's meant to be a no-alcohol evening; what have you really got to lose?'

When my children started at primary school, I began to feel really self-conscious turning up at the school gates each day. There was always one particular clique there and I never felt a part of it – it was like being back in the playground again. I felt a failure that I wasn't more popular. I would tell myself I was a bad mother – my daughter didn't enjoy as many play-dates as the other girls whose mothers were good friends. As soon as I got home, it was straight to the fridge for a glass of wine while my kids did their homework; a reward for getting through the pick-up and telling myself I deserved a break. Then that voice would start again: "This is a downward spiral, you're so weak, a mother who drinks," and so on.

Meg, 34

The mindfulness meditation exercises in 5:2 Your Worry (see pp.219–20) will help you become more aware that these thoughts aren't necessarily true or a part of you, that you have the choice to observe them and then simply let them pass.

I've used the mindfulness meditations to help me rationalise the situation, feel any negative thoughts, then let them go. I visualise my watershed hour, when I've eaten and I'm out of the danger zone. Maybe it's simple conditioning, but if I can make it to 9 p.m., I know I won't want a drink – I've done it, crossed the finishing line.

I think about how I'll just use my evening in a different way – catch up with my wife, read to the kids, check my diary, go online, ring a friend or family member. I see these as little rewards for staying off the booze. I also think about the health benefits of having two nights off and how much sharper I'll feel the next day at work. So when the next "drink night" comes round, it feels like a treat rather than a bad habit.

Robert, 34

Drinking and hypnotherapy

Foster's approach is to tackle our critical thinking via hypno-therapy, inducing a relaxed and yet conscious state to confront destructive thoughts with a more positive script.

I lie on a sofa in her consulting room with my eyes closed and the session begins. She addresses my inner critic, explaining that I don't have to believe all my negative assumptions but can choose to let them go, that I can feel safe and confident, say 'no' to a drink and enjoy my AFDs. Foster sends me a recording of our session and I replay it to reinforce those positive messages:

'Drift as much as you choose, as much as you'd like to. Notice how these two days a week off alcohol are full of good thoughts and feelings, the sensation of achieving something great for you. On these days, you will notice you feel calmer, safer, much more intuitive and creative, more optimistic.

'The day and night goes more quickly because you're not listening to your inner critic. Your mind and body are tuning in to that sensation of confidence, dealing with your life in a much healthier way. That intuitive, confident part of you is now your strongest voice. It is there to protect you and you realise your inner critic is just one voice, it's not the truth.

'Now when you do drink, you pick up a glass. You notice the glass, and the colour. You're noticing your wine so much more. You're more discerning about what you drink. AFDs are more fun, they're not about restriction.

Sometimes you drink, sometimes you don't. Whatever alcohol you choose, you're drinking it much more slowly. Other people drink faster than you, now you pace yourself. You're feeling proud that with each AFD you're building up a library of positive references.'

I listen to her recordings early on my two AFD evenings and the simple act of investing time, lying on my bed and focusing on her messages and my goals, does help to strengthen my resolve. Later that evening, I feel confident, relaxed and indifferent to an open bottle of wine in the fridge.

Ten ways to reduce your units, even on drink days

1) Try to cut out drinking before you eat, or, if you're out, make one light aperitif last until your meal. Start to associate drinking and eating as part of the same experience, not to be separated, at home or when you're out.

2) Be aware of 'mindless' drink habits – that glass of wine while you're cooking or watching TV. Check back on your list of when you drink and why; how many are 'mindless' and could be cut out or postponed until mealtime?

3) Alternate your drinks – for each beer, G&T or glass of wine, have a glass of water or a soft drink.

4) When you first start trying to drink less socially, keep it to yourself and stock up on white lies. Your drink buddies will resist any change in habit and may well try and dissuade you

– they'll encourage you to drink. Don't tell people you've cut back until you're confident of a shift in mindset. How would you find it easiest to explain why you're not drinking this evening? List some reasons and keep them at the back of your mind, for example,'I can't face a drink after going out last night,' 'I'm on antibiotics' or 'I've got to get up really early tomorrow.'

5) In the pub or at a social event, sip slowly and make your drink last – top up white wine with fizzy water or go for a low-alcohol beer. Sit a round out – but keep a glass in your hand. Reassure yourself that once your friends have had a couple of drinks, they won't notice what you're drinking. Be sure to buy the drinks when it's your round, though!

6) Delay your first drink by fifteen minutes every week. We all have that internal 'respectable' hour, when we look at the time and think, 'It's OK now to have a drink.' Our 'wine-o'clock' hour was 6 p.m. at weekends, which we've successfully pushed back to 7.30 p.m. over six weeks, simply inching it forward by fifteen minutes each week.

7) Keep on top of negative thoughts. 'It's been an exhausting day therefore I need a drink. I'll feel better tomorrow, that's when I'll give it a miss.' This is the inner critic looking to sabotage, so try to counter with a positive 'I have a choice. This feeling or thought won't last very long. In five minutes, I'll feel fine and the craving will pass.'

8) Sip, don't gulp, and put your drink down; be aware of trying to surf that automatic reflex to pick your drink up, and consciously leave it an extra minute or so. Build up to making one drink last an hour. Start with a twenty-minute time limit and graduate from there over two or three weeks.

9) Drink something different – if white wine slips down like water, then switch to something you know you can sip and savour. I usually steer clear of red wine because, even though I like the taste, it can make me feel heavy-headed after one glass. For this reason, it's my choice on one or two of my drink days because I know I'll be more moderate and cautious (and it's even better now I know that a little red wine can be good for you, especially if it contains the Tannat grape – see Drink Facts, pp.56–8).

10) Be aware that your inner critic will be at its most vocal the evening after a day without alcohol. 'I really deserve an extra few drinks tonight, I've proved I can do a few AFDs, so why not let my hair down?' Two or three AFDs only work in combination with relatively sensible drinking on other nights; otherwise you can find yourself slipping into a yo-yo pattern of abstaining then bingeing.

6 Don't forget the benefits

Remind yourself of the key 'wins' for you when you successfully 5:2 Your Drink. Keep them in mind to stay committed to your goals. 'Why do you want to change your behaviour?' asks Cornett. 'When you're tempted, that's when your motivational factors need to kick in; for example, I know I'll be more productive, proud when I wake up the next day, feel better in front of my children.'

On the 5:2 diet, weight loss and maintenance is the primary incentive that carries you through a fast day, but what about alcohol? You may experience a similar physical urge to satisfy your craving, so you need to know exactly why you're committed.

Take a pen and paper and write a list of the top five benefits of sticking to at least two AFDs each week, and being sensible for the other four or five.

Think of your own, but the following are worth bearing in mind:

- To rest my liver, giving it a forty-eight-hour window to rejuvenate and reducing my risk of liver disease.

- To lose weight.

- To feel more productive after a two-day alcohol break.

- To feel more energetic and alert.

- To save money.

- To feel like a better role model in front of my children.

- To feel the satisfaction of finally changing my attitude and shifting a habit.

There always used to be a justification to have a drink. I saw alcohol as a treat, a reward and a comfort. If I'd had a bad day, I deserved a drink, and if it was good, I had a drink to celebrate. Sometimes the excuse was feeble – "It's Friday," or even "There's an open bottle of wine in the fridge." But now I say to myself, since I've started the 5:2 routine, 'I don't want to drink every day.' I really didn't; I'd become sick of it and that was my main motivation. But that simple mantra has helped me resist. I also imagine and look forward to the virtuous feeling I have the next day – especially if my partner gives in to temptation.

Ed, 38

5:2 your liver

If the 5:2 Drink Diet can deliver you one great health benefit, it's resting your liver for forty-eight hours. Here's why it helps. Professor Chris Day, liver specialist at University of Newcastle and medical advisor to Drink Aware says, 'The main benefit from not drinking two days a week is psychological. It's much easier to say to yourself "I'm not drinking at all today," rather than "I'll only have one glass instead of two." If you have two days off a week you're more likely to drink fewer units overall. And less likely to make up for it on your drinking days – good news for your liver.'

We know that alcohol is harmful to the liver and there are two theories as to why.

1) When the liver breaks down alcohol, the process generates free radicals. These can cause oxidative stress leading to inflammation and scarring.

2) Alcohol makes our gut wall more permeable, allowing the bacteria living there to enter our blood stream, which goes directly to our liver.

Alcohol is a toxin and the risk of damaging your liver goes up incrementally – i.e. two drinks are worse than one. If you take 100 people who are drinking seven or eight units a day, 10 per cent will get serious liver disease.

You can spend twenty years damaging your liver and not know about it – drinking a couple of 175ml glasses of wine a day if you're a woman, or four pints of lager for men, is likely to bring on a condition called 'fatty liver', where your liver is overloaded and unable to process fat properly, causing abdominal pains and nausea. Continuing to drink heavily then leads to cirrhosis and liver failure.

The reason hangovers are so painful is that the liver normally produces glucose at night to provide energy to survive. Alcohol stops the liver doing that, so we wake up hypoglycaemic – with low blood sugar – making us feel dizzy and confused and craving fatty, sugary food and drinks. On top of that we're dehydrated, sweaty and flushed, as alcohol is a vasodilator: it makes blood vessels bigger.

There are three risk factors for your chance of developing liver disease: your genetic predisposition, being a heavy drinker and – the one many people don't know about – being overweight. Alcohol and obesity is a toxic combination for the liver – a good reason to 5:2 both alcohol and food.

7 Savour your drink

Alcoholic or nonalcoholic, taking time over your drinks will give you an opportunity to appreciate them both for different reasons and in different ways. Savouring a wine or beer on your drink days will help you to pace yourself and view alcohol in a different way.

'Really appreciate each glass rather than gulping it back,' says Foster. Enjoy each drink for as long as possible and be aware of your senses in the moment:

- Touching: feel the glass in your hand and the weight of it.

- Seeing: look at the glass and the drink with full attention and engagement, exploring every aspect of it.

- Smelling: hold it under your nose and really think about what you're noticing with each in-breath.

- Sipping and swallowing: how does it feel on your tongue, in your mouth? Think about the aftertaste and how you feel now, the instinct to taste it again.

Mark Williams, professor of clinical psychology at Oxford University, also advocates this approach. 'Rather than saying it's all about being a puritan, notice every single taste that's in your drink of choice. See if you can discern each ingredient. If you find you drink it too quickly, notice that feeling of "I've gulped it away and let myself down." Try not to judge yourself harshly, reset to zero and say, "I'll see if I can have another run at this"; the element of kindness here is the absolute hallmark of how you approach it.'

It's difficult at first to slow down and let myself focus simply on my drink; my mind is going a mile a minute, as usual, and I feel impatient. But I can see the merits of it – like eating and savouring my meal at the table instead of in front of the telly. I imagine myself to be a Zen-like person, composed and serene, and become aware that I do feel calmer.

Jane, 32

Repeat the exercise whenever you have a drink. Don't view wine, spirits or beer only as a means to an end – a sure way to get a high. Become a connoisseur – take a wine course, join a real-ale society; if you enjoy drink, appreciate its merits rather than viewing it as a way to escape.

As Foster says, 'Become more fussy about your drink and be more thoughtful. Avoid the three for two offer in your local supermarket.' Check wine columns in weekend supplements or online for good-value recommendations, read around your subject, think about quality rather than quantity.

At the weekend, instead of buying two bottles of wine for around £6 each, I buy one £12 bottle. It feels quite decadent, especially served in lovely glasses. Limiting how much alcohol there is in the house is a huge help – if it isn't there, I can't cheat.

Paul, 35

Going to a slighter smarter bar and ordering a glass of champagne was a lovely treat with a friend, rather than sharing a whole bottle at our local as usual.

Mary, 29

The same principles apply when enjoying nonalcoholic drinks, which should be regarded as a treat in themselves. 'Make up a nonalcoholic drink you really enjoy and spoil yourself,' says Williams.

Catherine Salway, founder of London's first alcohol-free bar, Redemption, and her mixologist Jayne Totty have created a selection of delicious 5:2 mocktails to enjoy on your AFDs, and to help reduce your units on a drink day too. 'What we've challenged ourselves to do with these mocktail recipes is to devise alternatives that won't make you feel deprived, creating drinks that are really adult with complex ingredients. They're nourishing but make you feel good too,' says Salway. You'll easily find the ingredients online and in supermarkets.

Take time preparing your mocktails and, if you can, make it a sociable activity – experiment with your partner or friend. 'Get the cocktail shaker out and the chips of ice and definitely use nice glasses. How you serve it is so important, it's about the theatre and the presentation,' Salway says. 'Make a conscious decision that this is what you'll do on your Drink Diet day, and that you want it to be a bit of an event.'

Experiment with different juices. 'Be an alchemist and try stuff out – good ones to keep in store are lemon, lime and pomegranate juice,' says Totty.

Look out for juices with health benefits, like beetroot. Endurance athletes often drink this before they race because it helps muscles use oxygen more efficiently. Studies have shown it can also help to reduce blood pressure.

'Try organic concentrated syrups too – lychee, agave, black cherry, goji, elderflower – and use them as a base. Don't forget herbs – think of each component of your drink; a sprig of mint can transform it. Invest in your ingredients, even if it's better-quality fizzy water', suggests Totty.

When Totty was first designing Redemption's menu she discovered that coconut water was an ideal substitute for vodka and gin. 'It's very hydrating, full of potassium and electrolytes.' It's also low in calories compared to coconut milk – a cup has around 45 calories. 'It's a vehicle for flavours, more viscose than water, and so it gives you a good base to build in other ingredients.'

All the recipes below make one full glass. Use a classic shot glass or an equivalent measure of 25 ml to get the quantity of the ingredients correct.

Cocorita

This mocktail version of a classic margarita nods to the tequila theme, using agave syrup in place of sugar syrup. Agave and tequila are both derived from the cactus plant.

> *Coarse salt*
> *1 lime wedge*
> *3 shots coconut water*
> *½ shot freshly squeezed lime juice*
> *½ shot agave nectar*
> *1 drop orange extract*
> *3–6 ice cubes*

- Spread the salt on a small plate and moisten the edge of a Martini or margarita glass with the lime wedge. Upend the glass onto the salt to create a salt rim.

- Fill a cocktail shaker or blender with the coconut water, lime juice, agave nectar, orange extract and ice, cover and shake or blend vigorously until well chilled and frothy.

- Strain the ingredients into the salt-rimmed glass and drink immediately.

Get creative and make a variety of margarita-inspired mocktails using different juices and infusions; simply replace a quarter of the coconut water with the juice or infusion of your choice.

Coco-politan

One for the *Sex and the City* generation, here is an alcohol-free version of that iconic drink; we like to think Carrie and gang would approve!

> 2 shots coconut water
> ½ shot cranberry juice
> ¼ shot agave nectar
> ¼ shot lime juice
> 1 drop orange extract
> 3–6 ice cubes
> A twist of orange peel

- Fill a cocktail shaker with the coconut water, cranberry juice, agave nectar, lime juice, orange extract and ice. Cover and shake vigorously until well chilled and frothy.

- Strain the ingredients into a Martini glass and drink immediately.

- Garnish with a twist of orange peel.

Rose and Elderflower Cooler

Elderflower is a classic English cordial, with the delicate perfumed notes of summer, enhanced further in this refreshing drink by a splash of rose water to create a classic wine-free spritzer.

3–4 ice cubes

1 shot organic elderflower cordial

A generous splash of rose water

Good-quality naturally sparkling mineral water

Edible flowers or a twist of lemon peel to garnish

- Pour the elderflower cordial and rose water into a tall glass filled with ice. Top up with sparkling mineral water and stir.

- Garnish with edible flowers or a twist of lemon peel.

Mockito

Punchy, refreshing and zesty, the art of 'muddling' your own mint and lime to create this iconic drink makes it special and still worth the effort, even without the rum.

1 lime, cut into eight wedges

10–15 fresh mint leaves

A good squeeze of agave nectar

4–6 ice cubes

Naturally sparkling mineral water

- Put the lime, mint and agave nectar into a sturdy highball glass and bash the mint and lime together using a muddler (or the end of a wooden spoon or rolling pin) in order to release the juices and essential oils from the lime and mint.

- Add ice and fill the glass with naturally sparkling mineral water.

Mauve Mary

Beetroot juice is sweet and earthy and offers a vibrant alternative to tomato juice; this makes a delightful twist to this brunch classic.

> *4–6 ice cubes*
> *A long stick of celery or cucumber*
> *¼ shot Worcestershire sauce*
> *¼ shot lemon juice*
> *2–3 drops of Tabasco*
> *5 shots beetroot juice*
> *A generous pinch of celery salt*
> *Slice of lemon to garnish*

- Fill a highball glass with the ice and add the celery or cucumber stick.

- Pour in the Worcestershire sauce, lemon juice and Tabasco and top with the beetroot juice; stir and serve topped with the celery salt and slice of lemon.

A Simple 5:2 Day Tokyo Iced Tea

Make this the night before your Drink Diet day and have a refreshing low-cal drink to enliven your afternoon. Green tea is rich in antioxidants and may even aid fat loss due to its thermogenic qualities.

- Make a large pot of green tea and leave to infuse for at least ten minutes.

- Pour into a large jug and add a few lemon slices and some fresh mint.

- Stir in some Xylitol or Stevia, available online or in some supermarkets, to sweeten to taste and leave in the fridge to infuse and chill. Serve over ice.

COMMON QUESTIONS

Why do I need to do this?

The 5:2 approach is ideal if your GP has suggested you should cut down on your alcohol intake, or you worry generally that you're too reliant on drinking at certain times and want to prove to yourself you can change an ingrained habit that's been part of your life for too long.

Which two days should I choose for my AFDs?

Unlike the other 5:2 life areas, your two AFDs should run together. This may be tricky if you wish to combine with a 5:2 diet where non-consecutive fast days are advised – ideally increase your AFDs to three in a row so that you're not dieting on the middle day but getting the benefit of being alcohol-free for more than one day at a time.

What should I bear in mind for the other five days?

The benefits of your two AFDs will naturally permeate your drink days too. You will start to realise that alcohol isn't that crucial to relaxation and pleasure, and you will unconsciously drink less most other days too.

Relish your drinks – alcoholic and nonalcoholic. Remind yourself this isn't a dramatic shift but a moderate tweak. As psychotherapist Philippa Perry says in 5:2 Your Relationship, 'Don't get too obsessional about it.' That's the point of every 5:2 life area – it's not extreme; it's comfortable and feasible.

Which other 5:2 life areas combine well with my AFDs?

 Any 5:2 life area that involves a new activity and doing something different will work well with AFDs. Think of

occasionally combining AFDs with your 5:2 **Relationship** days, because it's better not to drink when you're trying out some of the shared exercises. However, it's fine to have a drink to hand when you're doing some of the fun quiz-based steps or on a date night! You could think of doing your 5:2 **Drink** Diet alongside your **Fitness** plan too – reward yourself with a mocktail after a workout. Or perhaps consider timing your AFDs to coincide with 5:2 Your **Productivity** for an efficiency boost.

To feel smug and remind yourself how much money you can save on your 5:2 Drink Diet, combine it with 5:2 Your **Finance**. Start by jotting down your alcohol reduction overall and price it up.

Here's what mine looked like:

Me: Three days not drinking white wine is roughly a
    bottle and a half of wine per week = £13
Husband   = same saving
Monthly saving   = £104

Open a savings account for a few months and, as your AFDs accrue, so will this. Plan a weekend away, with no AFDs, as a further incentive.

DRINK FACTS

Unit Guide	
Small glass of red/white/rosé wine (125 ml), ABV 12%	1.5 units
Standard glass of red/white/rosé wine (175 ml), ABV 12%	2.1 units
Large glass of red/white/rosé wine (250 ml), ABV 12%	3 units
Lower-strength lager/beer/cider (1 pint), ABV 3.6%	2 units
Higher-strength lager/beer/cider (1 pint), ABV 5.2%	3 units

Unit Guide	
Bottle of lager/beer/cider (330 ml), ABV 5%	1.7 units
Can of lager/beer/cider (440 ml), ABV 4.5%	2 units
Alcopop (275 ml), ABV 5.5%	1.5 units
Single small shot of spirits (25 ml), ABV 40%	1 unit

Calorie Guide			
Wine	**Red**	**White**	**Rosé**
Calories in a 125 ml glass of wine	112	92	106
Calories in a 175 ml glass	158	130	149
Calories in a 250 ml glass	225	185	212
Beer and Cider	**Beer**	**Lager**	**Cider**
Calories in a pint of 3.6%	187	182	233
Calories in a pint of 5.2%	256	227	239
Calories in a 330 ml bottle of 5%	152	132	116
Calories in a 440 ml can of 4.5%	172	180	167

Alcopop	
Calories in a 275 ml bottle of 5%	192

Spirits (40%)	
Calories in a single shot (25 ml)	56

- The government's daily guidelines are 3–4 units for men and 2–3 for women, although Professor Chris Day, liver specialist at the University of Newcastle and medical advisor to Drink Aware, recommends two days off each week as well.

- On the plus side, a recent Spanish study found that drinking can reduce depression. The research followed 5,500 moderate drinkers, men and women, over seven years, and found that those who drank between two to seven glasses of wine a week were less prone to depression than non-drinkers. The findings were still significant when factors such as smoking, diet and marital status were taken into account.

- Although heavy drinking is associated with an increased risk of breast cancer, a new study has found that light to moderate consumption appears to have little effect on women's risk. The research included over 13,000 women between the ages of 20 and 91 and was conducted by the Centre for Alcohol Research at the National Institute for Public Health in Denmark.

- Scientists agree on the existence of an ingredient in red wine that, when drunk in moderation, can help to protect the heart, reduce 'bad' cholesterol and prevent blood clots. The Tannat grape, grown in south-west France as well as Uruguay, appears to offer the most benefits: it contains high levels of procyanidins – a class of flavanols found in plants, fruit and cocoa beans – that are likely to be behind the health-giving properties.

- The downside of excessive drinking is that liver disease is now the fifth biggest killer in the UK, according to the Department of Health, with the number of people dying from it rising by 20 per cent over the past decade.

- At least 13,000 cancers in the UK every year are the result of people's drinking habits. The research, carried out across eight European countries including the UK, has found that thousands of cancers could be prevented if men had the equivalent of no more than two drinks a day and women had no more than one.

5:2

YOUR
FITNESS

LIFE BEFORE MY 5:2 FITNESS PLAN

Exercise was always something other people did, or bored me about. When they weren't running a 10k, completing a duathlon at dawn or cycling to Oxford (OK, I'm referring to my husband here and not my imaginary friends) they, or rather he, were eulogising about the natural endorphin highs and the afterglow of achievement. Not to mention how much better he felt, and looked. I was mystified by such a dramatic change in attitude, a little irritated even, probably because I knew he was right. As you enter middle age, you can't ignore the research any more – the one factor that uniformly appears to lessen our chances of so many critical conditions – including high blood pressure, heart disease, obesity, cancer, even Alzheimer's – is regular exercise, even better if it's high intensity and cardiovascular (see Fitness Facts, pp.88–9, for recent studies).

It wasn't as if I hadn't tried to embrace exercise before. Over the years I'd sweated it out in Step and Zumba classes, stretched and 'omed' in yoga and cried with boredom in my local gym. None held any long-term appeal and all of them would lead me back to square one, demotivated, poorer and still relatively sedentary.

Then I discovered running. Over a year later, I'm still hooked. I love the immediate gratification of feeling my heart race by the time I reach the end of my street, the sense of anticipation and escape ahead of me as I hit my pace with the help of an inspiring playlist for an early morning run by the river.

There's no real epiphany here – I haven't run marathons around the world, transformed my body or changed my life as a consequence. I don't feel emotional or evangelical about running but, even so, I'm surprised how much I do enjoy it. In my own languid, low-key, anti-exercise-by-nature way, I'm a convert.

MAKING THE 5:2 CONNECTION

As much I enjoy running, however, it has gradually become more time-consuming. I've begun to feel guilty if I don't manage to run my route, which usually takes around an hour, four times a week. Factor in another ten or fifteen minutes for a warm-up and cool-down, and it was becoming a high-maintenance routine, everything that running promised not to be.

That's when I started reading about the rise of something called 'the minimalist workout', reported on by, among others, the *New York Times* columnist Gretchen Reynolds. In these workouts, sports scientists were pushing the boundaries, not of how much we exercise we should be achieving, but of how little. Who doesn't want to do less? This approach involves High-Intensity Interval Training (HIIT), a workout that alternates extreme bursts of high-intensity with short rests between.

The Tabata way

Professor Izumi Tabata helped to pioneer the HIIT workouts devised today with a study in 1996 in which Olympic speed-skaters were given a brief but punishing regime: cycling intensely for twenty seconds on stationary bikes, resting for ten seconds, repeated eight times for four minutes. After six weeks the results were significant. They had improved their anaerobic capacity by 28 per cent and their VO2 max – a measure of aerobic and cardiovascular power – by 15 per cent.

But this is about extreme effort – no compromise. It's brief but also incredibly gruelling. Tabata says that if you feel fine after this exercise that you haven't pushed yourself sufficiently. By the last two repetitions, it should feel incredibly challenging. He also believes, crucially for the 5:2 ratio, that completing this protocol twice a week, half the time outlined in his original study, can still offer real health benefits.

Ten years later, in 2006, Martin Gibala, a physiologist, and his colleagues at the McMaster University in Ontario, showed in a study that three minutes on a stationary bike – thirty seconds of all-out exertion followed by a few seconds' rest, then repeated – provided the same health benefits as a more moderate bike ride lasting up to 120 minutes.

More recently Professor Jamie Timmons, chairman of systems biology at the University of Loughborough, devised a three-minute workout involving a warm-up on an exercise bike for two minutes, followed by three all-out twenty-second bursts at maximum effort with a short rest between each one. Measurable health benefits were reported, including significantly improved insulin sensitivity (up to 24 per cent in two weeks), which can also help to protect against Type 2 diabetes.

Feel the pain for a bit of gain

In *The Fast Diet*, co-author and medical journalist Dr Michael Mosley refers to the theory of hormesis, where a small amount of stress can make you more resilient. He makes the valid point that the activities that feel uncomfortable, difficult, stressful – high-intensity interval exercise and intermittent fasting, to name but two – are often the ones that actually benefit us. The very discomfort we experience is what helps us 'repair', build cells and make us stronger. He includes the example of bitter vegetables – the reason they taste that way is because they contain chemicals that could be dangerous were they at higher levels. As it is, their low-level presence triggers stress responses, activating genes that repair. Vaccination is another example – where an inactivated or weakened form of a pathogen is introduced to the body, stimulating the immune system to create antibodies.

In terms of fitness, pushing ourselves that bit further, and it only has to be briefly, is what precipitates that 'repair' process. 'If you don't achieve "overload",' explains personal fitness trainer Steve Mellor, 'you won't adapt, and your body needs that stimulus for it to change. When you train, you have microtraumas in your muscle fibres, that feeling in your legs when they're painful and they ache afterwards. They are the tiny rips and tears in your muscle, stimulating recovery that will make it stronger.'

According to the most recent research (see Fitness Facts, pp.88–9), spending a few minutes each week at an all-out level of effort will give you at least the same benefits as moderate exercise over a longer time period and, best of all, the protocol can be adapted to many types of exercise – running, cycling, circuit training or swimming; anything where a sprint and a rest can be included. Since it's so intense, you can cut the time and frequency of your normal routine – no need to work out for so long. Combining this with the 5:2 ratio seemed like a winning formula.

I approached sports scientist and head of personal training and nutrition at Freedom2Train, Steve Mellor, who incorporates short, simple but tough and intense intervals into his workouts. He is enthusiastic about matching the 5:2 ratio with the HIIT protocol. 'Two days a week is a good amount of time to see and feel the benefits. It's putting a plan into place that's realistic. If you can't do two days a week, then you need to ask yourself why. I tell clients that if Barack Obama can manage to exercise every day, you can certainly do it twice a week.'

Consistency is key with any form of exercise and, since the 5:2 is a moderate ratio, it gives you the best chance of hitting your weekly target, however busy you may be.

As *Guardian* columnist Zoe Williams said when she tested out the 5:2 approach to fitness, 'If you want to know whether the two-day-a-week principle works, it does; even that frequency is habit-forming. It creates other healthful habits: I started making ridiculous snacks for myself – dainty asparagus spears on rye bread – as if trying to tempt into appetite an invalid from the royal family. The sense of being rationed makes you work harder, and for longer, and makes it all feel like less of a chore.'

Professor John Brewer, director of sport at the University of Bedfordshire says, 'In many ways the 5:2 model of exercise is the most practical. The two biggest barriers to exercise is time and cost. If you can in some way incorporate exercise into your life, rather than force a gap, you're more likely to succeed. You could argue that exercising at weekends – we call this group the 'weekend warriors' – is a natural 5:2 fit. I've slipped into this category. Use Saturday and Sunday to catch up on exercise, and that's your benchmark.'

Maureen MacDonald, a professor of kinesiology at McMaster University, also believes HIIT and 5:2 combine well. She recently researched a gentler interval practice compared to their original study in 2006, involving two different exercise training programmes for patients who'd been diagnosed with coronary artery disease.

Participants in the McMaster routine would warm up for five minutes, then cycle stationary bicycles at about 90 per cent of their maximum heart rate for one minute, followed by a minute for recovery. This was repeated ten times in succession and followed by a five-minute cool-down and lasted for a thirty-minute session. The second group completed thirty to fifty minutes of moderate intensity cycling exercise. In three months, they discovered a dramatic improvement in both groups, even though they had only completed the routine twice a week. 'Typically, you see, HIIT is superior to moderate intensity,' says MacDonald.

The 5:2 ratio wasn't something they'd planned on, she admits. They originally aimed for two days in the studio followed by one day at home. In reality, none of the participants completed that third day – somehow it felt like too much. So they settled for twice a week. 'If you're looking for evidence that it works two days, it did – clinically the most significant improvement was aerobic fitness. Two days fitted in with their life. It's not what we wanted when we started out, but in the end it worked.'

MacDonald also draws another comparison with HIIT and the 5:2 ratio – that to change the body, she says, requires a short, sharp shock, which is as good as something more frequent but less taxing.

'It seems that to get the body to adapt, we only need to make tiny changes within cells. But you need enough of a wake-up call. Inside the cells we have genes that determine the proteins we make and therefore the function of these cells. Depending on the signals the genes get, they regulate how much muscle you build, how much fat you will store.' Crucially, exercising at a lower level doesn't seem to change those signals as much as higher intensity exercise.

'I think you have to hit it with a hammer, which is the cohesive idea of 5:2,' says MacDonald. 'To wake up the metabolism of the cells we need to dramatically change them, really challenge them two days a week.'

Most surprising of all, perhaps, she discovered that it was the less fit participants who found it easier to 'hit the ceiling' for a short time each week, really push themselves hard, than exercise gently for longer.

'It's the reversal of what you'd think,' says MacDonald. 'That the less healthy should start slow. We found that wasn't the case. In other words, the human body can adapt to two, three, or even six or seven minutes of more intense exercise, compared to half an hour of strenuous but lower intensity.'

THE 5:2 FITNESS PLAN; aims and benefits

- HIIT is intense and challenging but it also feels a bit like cheating – little input for a large gain.

- HIIT can continue to burn calories up to forty-eight hours after you exercise. Following HIIT, your excess post-exercise oxygen consumption (EPOC), a measurably increased rate of oxygen intended to erase the body's 'oxygen' deficit, raises your metabolic rate.

- HIIT can reduce appetite and stem hunger pangs, according to research in the *International Journal of Obesity*, published in summer 2013. When they studied a group of exercisers, the ones who had completed very high-intensity workouts consumed the fewest calories afterwards.

- A realistic time commitment – perfect for people who struggle to exercise frequently or, like me, want to streamline one activity that they enjoy, e.g. running, making it shorter but more intense.

- When the going gets tough, and it should do, reassure yourself that it's extremely brief – it may hurt now but it will finish in five minutes, then you can forget about it for at least another two days.

- Expect your body to change – this level of aerobic activity will make you look more toned and feel more supple too.

- You will also learn how to combine 'incidental exercise' with everyday tasks on your other five days, increasing the effects of your two-day workouts.

GETTING STARTED ON THE 5:2 FITNESS PLAN

There is a choice between two HIIT workouts for your two fitness days – you can start with the shorter four-minute one and try the seven-minute one the following week.

Try alternating the two or, if you prefer, adapt the interval protocol to your existing exercise routine. For the ultimate 5:2 fitness regime, mix and match HIIT sessions twice a week with the incidental activity outlined in Step 6, which will hopefully change your daily habits – and find out in Step 7 why music will help you achieve and enjoy all these goals.

SEVEN STEPS TO MAKE THE 5:2 FITNESS PLAN WORK FOR YOU

1 **Is the 5:2 HIIT approach right for me?**
The intensity of HIIT routines can seem daunting, particularly if you don't exercise regularly, but they are easy to modify for any level of fitness. Start at a slower pace if you wish and build up gradually, and, for the first week or two, only choose the exercises that appeal to you. If the circuits seem too brutal at first, adapt the protocol to whatever workout you currently enjoy – be it swimming, cycling, running or working out at the gym – more on this in Step 5.

Make sure you're doing the exercises correctly and within your limitations, and be realistic about your base level of fitness. 'We do recommend you get clearance from your physician first,' says Chris

Jordan, director of exercise physiology at the Human Performance Institute in Florida. 'With our seven-minute workout, we also advise that beginners start slowly, take longer to complete each one and to recover between intervals.'

If you're a complete beginner, ideally book a personal trainer for just one session of HIIT to guide you through and give you advice for when you exercise alone. A one-off hour with a personal trainer is still substantially cheaper than the gym or regular aerobics and yoga, a small investment to get the most out of these exercises in the long-term.

In her recent research where participants were less healthy, MacDonald was strict about who could and couldn't do the HIIT training. 'I would say go to your doctor and make sure there aren't any other factors to consider. We didn't allow anyone with uncontrolled diabetes or angina in our study.'

She adds, 'We do highlight that we make the same recommendations as any other type of exercise too – do a warm-up and a cool-down.'

Bear in mind that it's during the post-exercise period that problems are more likely to occur, says MacDonald. 'When you're at rest, a different branch of the nervous system is regulating your heart-rate – it's like passing the baton, when your heart is between phases.' Avoid stopping abruptly, but bring your body back to its normal place gradually with a good warm-down.

I do stationary cycling interval training for twenty minutes first thing in the morning when I wake up (I set the alarm thirty minutes earlier than usual) and it really enlivens me for the day ahead. I combine it with a ten-minute warm-down afterwards and a mindful meditation [see 5:2 Your Worry, p.219], *and that seems to focus my thoughts to help tackle the day's myriad challenges ahead. I reward myself with a healthy breakfast – granola with blueberries and Greek yoghurt. Plus a large glass of beetroot juice.*

Ben, 42

2 Set goals

Now you've read about the benefits and realities of intense interval training, think about what you want to achieve by practising them regularly. What appeals to you most? How you'll look and feel? The long-term health benefits? Write a list of five reasons you really want to stick to the 5:2 Fitness Plan. We know that the physical and fitness gains are dramatic but, in the midst of your second circuit of twenty seconds of lunges or ab crunches, it may help to visualise them to keep you going!

Here's what my top three looked like:

1) Post-exercise high: I really like the way these exercises make me feel around fifteen minutes after my warm-down – unusually energised and lively, and the effects last for around three or four hours. That's the memory I cling on to, mid-Tabata sprint.

2) Brevity: I love how short these exercises are – I don't even need to set my alarm early to complete my seven-minute workout, which I can do on the kitchen floor before I get the children's breakfast going. The brevity more than makes up for the pain and intensity. When it gets gruelling, I can remind myself that this is a fair price for a routine that will be over so quickly.

3) Lean and mean: 'The crunches and lunges help build and maintain your muscle and lean mass,' explains Chris Jordan. 'You'll see more muscle definition.' Maybe he's got a point.

Within a month my upper arms look perkier, less like my daughter's pummelled Play-Doh; no anxiety about bingo wings when I wear my sleeveless dress is the best incentive there is.

And here are the top five goals of Catherine, 48:

1) To drop two dress sizes so I can fit into my wedding dress next May. When I don't feel like exercising, I think about it straining at the seams. Also, I visualise our first dance and imagine my husband's hand resting on my bulges as we dance in full view of the critical in-laws.

2) To sleep better – I'm a chronic insomniac so I'm hoping regular exercise will help cure that. My permanent exhaustion also explains why I overeat – I feel I need the calories just to stay awake.

3) To have a more varied lifestyle – if I get fitter I can join in with friends' adventures such as walking Hadrian's Wall or going coasteering.

4) Fitting into a wetsuit without feeling like a walrus. Wetsuits are the most unforgiving of garments but I want to zip one up without feeling like I'm a laughing stock.

5) Be someone my children look up to and want to emulate. My parents were overweight and not very active when I was growing up and as a result I too favour a sedentary lifestyle. I want to break out of that for my children's sake.

The incentives I use to encourage myself are imagining "the new me" – healthy, active, slim, energetic. I also try not to make

*deals with myself such as "If Hester doesn't go to Aquafit then
I don't have to either" – I make myself go anyway. Exercise
classes that you have to pay for in advance are good too –
I've already spent the money so it's a waste not to go.*
    Catherine, 48

3 The four-minute 5:2 workout

Devised by Steve Mellor, this four-minute 5:2 workout incorporates the Tabata principle. He advises twenty seconds of one of the exercise types listed below, followed by resting for ten seconds, then performing twenty seconds of another exercise, resting for ten seconds, then returning to the first exercise and repeating for a total of four minutes of all-out effort. These are ideal to practise indoors or, as we did, in a local park.

Warm up for ten minutes, stretching from head to toe and, if you're outside, running with fast bursts. After your four minutes of intense exercise, warm down for five minutes, stretching more slowly and deeply from head to toe. To build up further, you can take a longer rest of ten minutes after your first four-minute block, and then repeat once more for an eight-minute workout. There are also some suggested variations below.

Total exercise time: four minute workout with maximum effort and short rests; fifteen minutes' stretching. Time yourself with a wrist watch or a mobile phone.

Here are the seven different types of exercises you can alternate in your four-minute burst:

1) **Burpee** – Assume a full press-up position with your hands and toes on the ground, your body forming a straight line from feet to head. Keep your head looking down but do not bend at the neck. Jump your feet up towards your hands,

getting them as close as possible. Stand up and jump up with your hands above your head.

2) **Mountain Climber** – Assume a press-up position on your toes and hands. Make sure the body is in one straight line from head to toe. Drive one knee up towards the chest as quickly as you can then change legs. This movement mimics running and blasts the core!

3) **The Get-Up** – Starting in a press-up position, bring your right foot up to the outside of your right hand and stand up, pushing through the heel of your right foot. Jump back into the press-up posiiton and repeat on the other side, making sure you squeeze your glutes as you stand up.

4) **Squat** – Stand with your feet about shoulder-width apart and your arms out straight at shoulder height. From there reach back with your hips and, bending your knees, lower them down towards the ground as if you are about to sit down in a chair. As you lower down, make sure you keep your knees pushed out in line with your toes so that you fire up your glutes and protect your knees. Stand up as fast as you can and repeat. Keep the core engaged while squatting.

5) **Walking Lunges** – Stand with feet shoulder-width apart and knees facing forwards. Raise your right leg to hip level, bending your knee to ninety degrees and step forward into a lunge so that both knees are bent at a ninety-degree angle. Alternate right and left legs. Make sure you keep your feet apart when lunging, this helps hit the glutes and free up the hips. Imagine you are on train tracks.

6) **Plank Push-Up** – Assume a plank position by lying face down on the floor, placing your elbows and forearms on the ground

and elevating your body so that weight is supported on balls of the feet and by the elbows (bent to ninety degrees) and forearms. Your body should form a straight line. Don't allow the hips to drop. Push up onto the right hand, then the left. Then lower the right hand back to the elbow and forearm and the left hand back down so that both elbows and forearms return to the floor. Repeat.

7) **Squat Press** – Assume a squat stance, as if about to sit on a chair, with a Theraband (a broad strip of stretchy tubing) running around and under both feet. Your hands should be up and next to your shoulders. From there, lower your bottom towards the ground and bend your knees. Make sure you keep your knees pushed out in line with your toes to protect them. Stand up as fast as you can and extend your arms up straight and lock out the elbows. Lower the hands back down to the shoulders and repeat. You don't have to use a Theraband but it helps to fire up the muscles with extra resistence and maintain a good body position.

Here are five examples of how you can mix and match:

1) Do as many get-ups as you can in twenty seconds, rest ten seconds. Then do as many squat presses as you can in twenty seconds and rest again for ten seconds. Then back to the get-ups and so on, for a total of four minutes.

2) AMRAP – 'as many rounds as possible' – choose two to three exercises from the list above and perform ten reps of each exercise to complete one set. Do this repeatedly for four minutes resting for a few seconds between sets if required. Count how many sets you perform.

3) Do walking lunge ten reps, squat press ten reps and mountain climber ten reps, moving as fast as you possibly can. Try to get through as many rounds of each of those sets in four minutes, resting for a few seconds between sets if needs be.

4) Choose three exercises to fill your four minutes; perform twenty reps of each exercise to complete one set. Try to complete four sets in total and time yourself so that you can aim to beat it next time. No resting in between.

5) Burpee twenty reps, squat twenty reps, plank push-up twenty reps. Get through this set as fast as you can then repeat, ideally, another three times. Stop the timer at four minutes regardless.

My first four-minute HIIT circuit

I meet Steve Mellor in the park where my four-minute workout will take place. After a thorough warm-up, as described above, we start with a gruelling round of squat presses, plank push-ups and walking lunges alternated with burpees, mountain climbers and squats. Although he explains to me about the intensity of these exercises, I'm still quite shocked how challenging such a short routine can be. Within minutes I feel convinced I won't be able to complete the circuit – sweating, out of breath, giddy and faint. Time distorts: the ten-second rest time goes in a blink, the twenty-second exertion seems to last an eternity.

By the last round, I am floundering and fatigued; my limbs are like lead. Mellor coaxes me like a midwife, firm but encouraging, 'Come on, not much longer, we're nearly there. Keep going – stronger now. All out now – only a couple of minutes to go,' and I can't help thinking that this is only mildly less strenuous and challenging than my last childbirth. Then, thankfully, something kicks in, maybe the endorphins, and I summon a last burst of energy, lunging deeper, pushing harder and kicking higher for that last twenty-second gasp. I feel euphoric that I've managed it and even jog back with Mellor across the park before a warm-down.

I can't believe it only took twenty minutes; the effects are like a ninety-minute run – my legs ache, as do my arms and muscles, bottom and upper thighs. I also feel energetic, not remotely exhausted, and get back determined to Tabata my workout that morning (see 5:2 Your Productivity).

I practice Mellor's workout three days later when my muscles have recovered, pleased that the 5:2 ratio allows me a decent amount of time to rejuvenate before giving it my all once again. It still feels tough but I enjoy completing them alone; I also feel I'm a step ahead, knowing how to achieve the best from each exercise thanks to a one-off personal training session.

My advice would be, if possible, share the exercises with a partner or friend, it can really motivate you. I enjoyed doing this workout with my husband, telling him what to do after I'd been through the circuit with my personal trainer. I admit not only was it satisfying to stand over him and bark orders,

"Quicker, higher", etc. it really helped to motivate him, and it was nice having someone there to watch and encourage me too. '

Jan, 48

4 The ultimate seven-minute workout

In summer 2013, Chris Jordan and Brett Klika, at the Human Performance Institute in Florida, published research in a scientific journal detailing a workout designed by Jordan for the time poor, aimed at business clients who spent their time travelling and staying in hotels. 'These twelve exercises were created with that in mind,' says Jordan. 'We used the research around HIIT to provide a combined workout of aerobic and resistance training that can be done just about anywhere with no equipment and in minimal time.'

The research has shown that even a few minutes at an intensity approaching your maximum capacity creates changes in muscle that can compare to several hours of normal, low or moderate-intensity cycling or running. The exercises should be performed as quickly as possible with little or no resting time between each one and there should be a fair level of discomfort. The payoff? A potentially very tough but very short workout. Jordan and Klika acknowledged in their research that the general population may not (or should not) attempt maximal-intensity exercise, but should aim to progress to twenty minutes of high-intensity (approximately 80–90 per cent of maximum heart rate) exercise.

- Perform each of the twelve exercises in succession for thirty seconds per exercise to complete one circuit. Repeat the circuit twice more for a total of three circuits, which should take around twenty minutes as a nonstop, high-intensity workout.

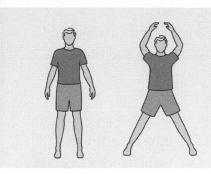
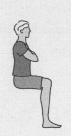

1 Total Body
Jumping Jacks

2 Lower Body
Wall Sits

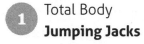
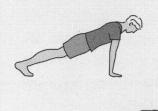
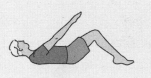

3 Upper Body
Push-Up

4 Core
Abdominal Crunch

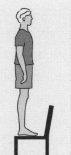
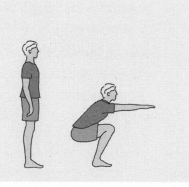

5 Total Body
Step-Up

6 Lower Body
Squat

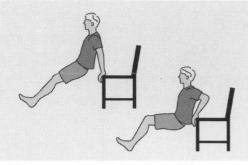
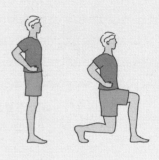

7 Upper Body
Tricep Dips

8 Core
Plank

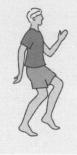
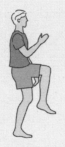

9 Total Body
High Knees

10 Lower Body
Lunge

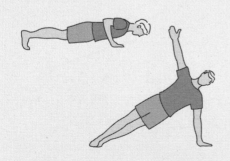

11 Upper Body
Push-Up & Rotation

12 Core
Side Plank

- Move from one exercise to the next with minimal (five to ten seconds) or no rest.

- Warm-up prior to the workout with dynamic stretching (for example, shoulder rolls, arm circles, leg swings, hip rotations, walking on the spot). Cool-down with stretches after the workout too.

Doing such intense exercise just twice a week doesn't make this workout seem like such a daunting prospect. It's over before you know it. I feel if I've got the self-discipline to do this, then it invigorates me and makes me physically and mentally prepared for the day ahead. It actually puts me in a good mood and fosters a really positive attitude, which is not bad for someone who isn't usually a 'morning person'. I'm also not a fan of gyms so this is a great – and free! – workout which can be done pretty much anywhere.

I also try and combine the two workouts with "productive days" [see 5:2 Your Productivity]. I get into work and I feel fully charged up, ready to steam into all the things that need to be done that day. On these days my mountains seem to become molehills.

Raj, 40

5 5:2 HIIT flexibility

The Tabata protocol is as versatile as the 5:2 ratio – it can combine with any other exercise discipline or routine that can be done at high intensity.

Circuit exercises

You can Tabata anything – press-ups, squats, rowing – as long as you can push yourself with the intensity of sprinting.

Cycling

Although it's easier to accelerate and rest on an exercise bike, a road bike is good too for a twenty-second burst – then slow down and rest your feet on the pedals for a ten-second break before repeating.

Running

If you're running, try a robust Tabata of thirty seconds with a ninety-second rest time. 'That thirty seconds must be flat out – think Usain Bolt, absolutely on your limit,' says Steve Mellor. 'Or you can push yourself for twenty seconds and rest for ten. Swing out those arms and legs as far as you can. Keep forcing the body to move that bit faster.' Push to your maximum. Then walk briskly for ninety seconds, and repeat for a total thirty-minute run. Don't forget a five-minute warm-up and cool-down.

I have now adapted my running routine, cutting it from an hour to half an hour and incorporating an HIIT protocol within it – as outlined by Mellor. My runs are more demanding and challenging: it's not as easy as it used to be, but then the pay-off is far greater. I feel I'm pushing myself and, best of all, I can confidently commit to forty minutes of exercise – including a warm-up and cool-down – twice a week. I feel more energetic, leaner and lither too.

Skipping rope

Perfect for a Tabata stretch – skip as fast as you can with intervals, either feet together or using the 'boxer shuffle', with alternating heels in front, and/or kick heels towards your bottom.

Swimming

A great non-impact exercise where you can alternate sprinting and resting up and down a pool, toning the upper arms as well as improving aerobic performance.

I have recently taken up kayaking in the local river and find I can pelt along for a good stretch at top speed – and an added bonus is that it impresses people on the riverbanks (until they see me gasping for breath down the river).

Tom, 36

6 Incidental activity

According to research (see Fitness Facts, pp.88–9), our rate of activity during the day is as key to our fitness levels as the formal exercise we manage to carve out each week. Non-exercise activity thermogenesis (NEAT) is physical movement during our daily lives that isn't planned or conscious – running up the stairs to brush our teeth when we're late, carrying heavy shopping bags, vacuuming, emptying the bins, even fidgeting. Those minute exertions that can make us wince, as we bend down to pick the remnants – peas, rice, soggy toast – of kids' teas glued to the kitchen floor, really make a difference to our metabolic rates. Particularly if we become more conscious of them and factor them in as assiduously as our HIIT workouts.

Medical journalist and author Dr Michael Mosley, also a big fan of HIIT, has said that he achieves his NEAT motion by getting up and having a walk around for every hour when he's working at his desk. He also cycles a mile and a half to the station every day, building his HIIT into his trip, and always takes the stairs instead of the lift.

Mixing and merging HIIT twice a week with incidental exercise is the perfect combination, as Mosley has discovered. 'That will be enough to see positive effects on your weight loss and also your health,' says Mellor. 'It's amazing how much fitter you can be if you build in incidental activity. Be conscious of taking a quick wander every hour if you're at work. Wear a pedometer and track how many steps you walk each day – 10,000 is an ideal.'

Five ways to boost your incidental fitness

1) Walk 10,000 steps each day – think of ways to increase those extra steps; walk up stairs and never take a lift.

2) Cycle or walk to work. Get off the train, bus or Tube a stop early and walk the rest of the way.

3) Tabata your housework for a powerful hit of incidental fitness – if you're cleaning your home, speed up for some of the activities. Give yourself a time limit and aim to increase your heart-rate with certain tasks like carrying the vacuum cleaner, emptying all the bins in the house or changing the beds. Put music on for added impetus – see Step 7.

4) Simply stand up more whenever you can, when you're on the phone or at work. People who sit for fewer than three hours a day live around two years longer than more sedentary peers, a paper published in 2012 in the online journal *BMJ Open* found.

5) When you watch TV, lengthen your legs, point your toes and then flex your heels, and repeat, to feel that stretch in your calves.

I decided to stop using my husband and children as my personal slaves. Whilst I'm watching television, if I want something to eat or drink, I have to get it myself. More often than not, I don't bother, so ironically my laziness means that I'm snacking less!

*I also set myself little missions during the ad breaks –
such as sort out the dirty washing and load the machine,
empty the dishwasher or decide what I'm wearing
tomorrow and lay it out. It helps me feel more organised
in the morning too.*

Steph, 47

7 Move to the music

There's no way round it, these exercises may be
quick, but they're punishing too. One proven way
to aid endurance and, crucially, boost pleasure while powering
through your lunges, squats or sprints is music.

Dr Costas Karageorghis, sports psychologist at Brunel
University, has spent the last twenty years focusing exclusively
on the special relationship between music and exercise, in
particular the psychophysical and ergonomic effects. More
recently he has been researching the effect of music on high-
intensity exercise, when you move from aerobic to anaerobic
(your body's ability to operate without oxygen) capacity or, as
Karageorghis puts it, 'The point where it feels really painful,
where you can feel acidosis in the muscles and a sharp increase
in the heart-rate.' In his studies he discovered that even at this
intensity, when it's assumed athletes and exercisers would be
beyond absorbing external stimuli like music, it does affect how
they feel – depending on what they listen to. 'Therein lies the
beauty of well-selected music', he says. 'It helps us to colour the
effects of fatigue, make exercise more bearable at the point that
you derive most physiological benefit from it.' In other words,
when you're most likely to want to give up.

According to Karageorghis, there are four aspects of music

that drive us: rhythm response, musicality, cultural impact and association.

The first two are internal – how our bodies react to the stimuli – and the last two relate to our emotional response – what an artist means to us, the impact and interaction of lyrics, memory and association.

Individual response is key in motivating us through difficult periods of exercise. 'If music is arbitrarily selected, the reduction of perceived exertion is 8 per cent,' says Karageorghis. 'If it's well selected, personally chosen, influenced by peer groups and friends, etc., the benefits are as great as 12 per cent.'

It's only when I try and exercise without my music that I realise how crucial a soundtrack is to my run or interval workout: if my iPad hasn't recharged in time, I can't run, simple as that. What music blocks out is as important as what it creates – without a soundtrack, I can feel my body straining, the blood in my ears and my heart beating, the slow thud of my feet on the pavement, my fallibility and imperfections. Music erases these flaws, makes me feel streamlined, super-fast, as if I'm starring in my own film.

Create your perfect playlist

Choose music with a relatively slow tempo to begin your workout and then slowly speed up the beats per minute – look out for apps that sync beats per minute with your playlists. Think about music that can transport you, physically and emotionally. Choose songs from your past with strong positive links and memories or film scores that have inspired you – the more personal the better.

'If you have high-tempo music, and all you have to do is switch it on and go with it, then it takes away the element of decision-making, which means you'll be more likely to achieve your goal,' says MacDonald.

'I look forward to listening to my current playlist as much as the run itself,' says Mellor. 'It's very emotive and picks you up. I say to clients, it's like appearing in your own little commercial, it envelops you in your own world. It can be a key feature in your motivation.'

Simon McEwen, runner and *Q* music magazine associate editor says, 'For me, a successful running playlist should be predominantly beat-driven, energetic dance music, with the odd euphoric pop tune thrown in to revive those tired legs. Ideally the tracks you choose should be quite long and similar-sounding; schizophrenic and erratic sequencing can interrupt your running flow. Nobody wants Captain Beefheart popping up on their shuffle, it will only throw your rhythm out. The trick is to create a seamless, unchallenging mix of upbeat sounds which make you want to dance – preferably in a forward direction! I find the following playlist ideal – it lasts for forty-five minutes but is also good for shorter runs or workouts.'

1) Movin' On Up – Primal Scream 3:48

   'A familiar, much-loved song which immediately makes me happy and gets me in the mood. I start walking fast to this to warm up, then begin jogging as soon as the handclapping comes in.'

2) Open Eye Signal – Jon Hopkins 7:48

   'This slow-building instrumental electronica track is ideal for gently upping my pace.'

3) Diane Young – Vampire Weekend 2:40

   'A jolt of upbeat euphoric pop keeps me on track. Though trying to run in time to the regimental drums is a challenge.'

4) I Feel Love (12-inch version) – Donna Summer 8:15
   'A running classic. The pulsating rhythm and Donna's ethereal vocals signal it's time to get in full stride now. Wish I hadn't chosen the long version though!'

5) Rez (2011 edit) – Underworld 6:02
   'More a frequency than a conventional dance track, this propulsive, euphoric techno provides a much-needed endorphin rush.'

6) The Throw (extended version) – Jagwar Ma 6:54
   'I'm flagging a bit now so the baggy groove of this keeps both my tempo and spirits up. When the bass line kicks in, I kick harder.'

7) Hannibal – Caribou 6:16
   'Gorgeous, fluid electro which chimes perfectly with my heavy breathing. Not far to go now.'

8) Deep Blue Day – Brian Eno 4:00
   'There's a weightlessness to this blissed-out ambient track which makes it ideal to warm down and stretch to. I concentrate on my breathing then bathe in the righteous afterglow of a good workout. Time for a lie-down.'

COMMON QUESTIONS

How will I feel when I do these exercises?

At the time, uncomfortable and possibly convinced you may not get through the sequence. As Steve Mellor says, 'If you can still talk while you're doing them, you're not going hard enough. You should be sweating, gasping for air, thinking to yourself, "I'm going too hard." Gradually these feelings will feel familiar, although they should always be there; as you get fitter you'll push yourself more to create the same intensity.'

What benefits can I expect to feel and see?

Within two or three weeks, depending on how hard you push yourself and how frequently you repeat your HIIT, you will see more overall definition.

Which other 5:2 life areas combine well with fitness?

Fitness is a perfect complement to every 5:2 life area, in particular:

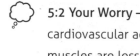 **5:2 Your Worry** – Dr Paul Jackson, fatigue specialist, says cardiovascular activity is best to induce a good night's sleep: muscles are less tense and endorphins also increase overall relaxation. Also ideal to try one of Professor Mark Williams's mindful meditations (see p.219) after a warm-down when the body is naturally relaxed.

 5:2 Your Finance – if you want to follow Step 4 and reduce your fixed costs by 10 per cent, then start with that pricey and underused gym membership. Exercise for free in or out of doors with Steve Mellor's exercises, or go for a run.

 5:2 Your Screen Life – do something different by exercising when you're on your digital detox, challenging your body and brain in a completely different way. Involve your children with a (much easier!) version of the HIIT workouts, or run while they cycle with you.

 5:2 Your Drink – keep yourself occupied with exercise. You'll be more likely to crave water than alcohol after an intense workout.

 5:2 Your Environment – cycle or walk instead of driving.

 5:2 Your Productivity – start the day with an HIIT and then apply the same technique to whizz through certain office or housework tasks.

What days should I do it on?

Ideally pick nonconsecutive days so the body can recover – any aching muscles will have repaired themselves within a day or two. However, for optimum fitness, don't leave it longer than two or three days between workouts because you can start to lose the benefits after this time. 'It's best to have the body in an elevated state of calorie burning for as long as possible, so a two-day gap is a good place to start,' says Mellor.

FITNESS FACTS

- HIIT training has been shown by several different studies to be effective because it produces molecular changes in the muscles similar to that produced after several hours of exercise. The key to these molecular changes is having intervals between the exercises – of ten seconds – and to be most effective you should alternate using the large muscles of the upper and lower body; so, for example, do press-ups followed by sprinting.

- Tabata's HIIT training is not only an excellent way to exercise but research has also shown that, when compared to other ways of exercising, it helps burn more calories when your workout has finished. Dr Tabata is due to publish further results that show that in the twelve hours following a Tabata workout, you burn 150 calories due to EPOC (excess post-exercise oxygen consumption), the increased rate of oxygen intake after exercise.

- As if you haven't seen enough evidence already, HIIT training has also shown to affect appetite. In a study at the University of Western Australia in Perth, following a bout of high-intensity exercise, participants consumed significantly fewer calories than after medium-intensity exercise.

- NEAT (non-exercise activity thermogenesis) plays a crucial role in the burning of our daily calorie intake, but sedentary lifestyles and reliance on technology is impinging on it. Dr James Levine, endocrinologist and author of *Move a Little, Lose a Lot*, estimates that what he describes as 'sitting disease' is to blame for between 1,500–2,400 calories per day not being used up in incidental exercise. One study published in the journal *Medicine and Science in Sports and Exercise* found that on average someone working in a sedentary job only takes 5,000 steps a day compared with 18,000 for a man in the Amish community.

- Choose when you exercise wisely. Feeling tired mentally shouldn't affect our physical performance, but research at the University of Kent has discovered that, despite our muscles still being up to the job, psychologically we feel less able to exercise and have less stamina after a hard day's thinking.

5:2

YOUR FINANCE

LIFE BEFORE MY 5:2 MONEY DIET

It seems I'm quite fond of letting money slip through my fingers. I can go for ages without buying anything, but I still dream about a time when I can – self-denial now with the promise of material paradise later on. As much as I challenge such a shallow notion, that inner reflex is still hard to resist: I'll be happier, I think, when I can buy a nicer bag so I don't have to carry my papers in a supermarket bag on the train; when I can buy a smarter sofa to replace the one that long ago lost the battle to three toddlers and numerous spillages; when I can buy a pastel-coloured food processor that is the culinary equivalent of a Fiat 500. I rarely get the chance to go shopping these days but still like the idea of owning, in no particular order, a rice cooker, a shed in the garden, a wireless printer, and a new winter coat.

The odd object of desire that I do manage to purchase never quite lives up to the anticipation. That bubble-gum-pink coat I yearned for is fine, nice, but not the candy-fuzz of happiness I dreamt it would be. Nor has the handheld vacuum cleaner, which now sits neglected under the sink as my husband told me it would do, quite lived up to expectations. The joy of spotless stairs and sucking up Cheerios cemented to the floor didn't last that long, surprisingly.

I remind myself of this, of course, as I click, flit and fly between Amazon, Topshop and Next online, sucked in by endless email alerts promising promo codes, free delivery, loyalty discounts. Harmless diversionary activities as long as I don't buy anything, I reassure myself, but the endless looking begins to feel furtive, empty, adding to that steady drip-drip of want, desire and disappointment, as well as wasting a colossal amount of time.

My children's shopping habits are increasingly shaped by the internet too, hooked in to ever more intrusive techniques – their devices squeak and vibrate with alerts to update this and buy that. They're invited to read about a pop star or actor, then click on a site where they can buy clothes just like theirs; I find myself stalked by personalised banner ads while I'm on other websites, reminding me of the products I nearly bought for myself or my kids but managed to resist. I can see the connection between screen time and consumerism, surfing from site to site, eternally restless and desiring something but never fully engaged or satisfied (see 5:2 Your Screen Life).

As well as being vulnerable to these developments, I'm also deeply fearful of having no money and fully identify with what writer Martin Amis has referred to as 'tramp dread' – the terror that if you stop working, you won't just fall overdrawn or behind on your bills but will end up on the streets. You'd think this ever-lurking fear of destitution and financial ruin would at least make me cautious and aware of where every penny goes. Sadly not. Instead I worry that we haven't got enough money to get us through the month, then get ambushed by a 20 per cent discount alert from the supermarket. I veer between fear and denial, in a haze about my personal finances and only brave enough to check my online account, through closed fingers, no more than once a month – heart sinking when I see, as I always do, that tell-tale capital D scrolling down my balance column. If anyone was in need of the short, sharp shock of 5:2 to my financial system, it was me. If it could be delivered in a twice-weekly dose in a relatively painless fashion, all the better.

MAKING THE 5:2 CONNECTION

I began to realise that of the many areas where the 5:2 ratio could have most impact, it would be money. Why? Because the gains are so appreciable. When you can hold the extra cash you've managed to save at the end of each week, or transfer it into a savings account, it's an obvious win.

Just like stepping on the scales the day after a week of fasting, or buckling your belt to the next notch, it's a visible gain that gives you instant incentive to keep going. There's nothing elusive or hard to measure about having more money left at the end of each week.

Also, like the 5:2 diet, it introduces an element of challenge imposed by a constraint that can often inspire creative thinking. There's nothing like 500 calories a day to make you more inventive – searching for ever-greater taste hits with chilli and garlic, coriander, lemon and lime. Slashing your spending budget for two days each week will make you similarly imaginative, creating benefits that you hadn't expected, including the fact that you'll be consuming less and gaining green points for the 5:2 Your Environment chapter, feeling more resilient and less manipulated by consumer advertising and sneaky online selling tricks, as well as being generally more independent, resourceful and able to amuse yourself for free. Those feelings of wellbeing and control are as satisfying when applied to your purse strings as to any other area of your life. And the practical benefits become clear to see too.

I approached Merryn Somerset Webb, financial advisor and editor-in-chief of personal finance magazine *MoneyWeek*, who felt it was a very manageable way forward. 'One day isn't enough to change your finances, but three is probably too much to focus on so intensely, so it's a good system. You should find your discretionary spending falls by 30 per cent over a week, and if you're capable of rolling that into a pension with a two-day money fast during your working life, you've made your non-working life significantly more comfortable.'

Professor Karen Pine, psychologist and co-author of the money makeover guide *Sheconomics* was also enthusiastic about the Money Diet's potential to alter habits. Pine, who specialises in Doing Something Different (DSD) as a behavioural change technique, can see that 5:2 is a powerful but also very realistic way of cultivating a new approach. 'To suddenly deprive yourself of something seven days a week feels impossible, and miserable, but this idea that the change is temporary and you always have that option to go back to how you were can have a lovely, subtle effect.'

THE 5:2 MONEY DIET; aims and benefits

- Tighten your purse strings today, with the built-in psychological comfort of knowing you can spend, within reason, tomorrow.

- Most spending plans fail because they're not realistic – this one is.

- Reduce daily spending twice a week and expect to save up to 30 per cent on your normal weekly budget.

- Overhaul your personal finances without living a life of austerity most of the time.

- Spending sensibly just some of the time will influence your behaviour a lot of the time.

- You will feel less anxious about money, less prone to impulse-buying and more secure about your financial future.

- You will be more self-aware, able to confront difficult money issues and understand your money motivations.

GETTING STARTED ON THE 5:2 MONEY DIET

These steps are a two-pronged attack, firstly to help you save money in the short term, but also to think about it more deeply in the long-term: spending nothing or as little as possible on your Money Diet days, but also using that time to think about your emotional connection with money.

SEVEN STEPS TO MAKE THE 5:2 MONEY DIET WORK FOR YOU

1 **Do a money audit**

It's crucial to know exactly what's coming in and going out of your account, where the spending leaks and hidden costs lie, and two days each week is more than enough time to take control of them.

This money audit will help initiate a new way of thinking about money, reducing anxiety by confronting your greatest financial fears while knowing that for the rest of the week you can relax. Just like the 5:2 diet, you may anticipate all those little treats you've denied yourself, but when it actually comes to it, that urge will feel curiously less urgent. Instead you'll be more moderate than you suspected you could be every day of the week.

Begin by taking a small notebook and a pen with you wherever you go – this is the only part of the Money Diet that does require a small daily commitment but, remember, you only have to complete this for a week or two at the most to record an invaluable snapshot of your spending life. Keep track of how much you withdraw from cash machines and where it goes, and hold on to receipts for cash purchases.

The more meticulous the better – don't round up costs; write down pence as well as pounds. Note the date and a brief description of the purchase, and how you paid. Pine recommends that you 'Try taking photos of everything you buy. It's something people do with food and they find that a visual record can be very powerful.'

Then, on your first Money Diet day, sit down and, on an A4 piece of paper, draw a line down the middle. Mark one side 'in' and the other side 'out'. Use the pointers below to help you. If you share your finances, do the exercise with your partner.

Money in

1) You and, if applicable, your partner's take-home salary and/or self-employed earnings after tax, and/or pension if you are drawing it.

2) Earnings from any other source (after tax) – include any income from property, trusts, dividends, even eBay earnings.

3) Child or any other benefits.

Money out

1) Mortgage or rent.

2) Direct debits and standing orders including savings, council tax, credit card payments, utility bills, memberships and mobile, internet and subscription services. Any yearly payments such as TV licence, home insurance, car tax and MOT – divide these by twelve and calculate a monthly figure for each one.

3) One-off or non-regular payments, i.e. car repairs, emergency plumber, new washing machine – calculate a monthly 'slush' fund for these types of costs.

4) Monthly living costs – food, drink, petrol, public transport, childcare, and also holidays (though you may view these as nonessential), birthdays and parties, Christmas.

5) Nonessentials – clothes, films, music, books, meals or drinks out, taxis, impulse purchases.

How the figures add up for Vicky, 24

Money in per month £2,100

Money out per month

1. Rent   £580
2. Direct debits   £450 (phones, utilities, TV, insurance,
                        council tax, gym membership)
3. One-off payments   £350 (car repairs, new toaster)
4. Living costs   £540 (food, drink, petrol)
5. Nonessentials   £360 (meals out, clothes, DVDs)

Total money out £2,280

Money out minus nonessentials £1,920

You should have three figures now:

a) Money in
b) Money out
c) Money out minus nonessentials

These are your three most important figures. If you're fortunate enough for a) – money in – to be higher than c) – money out minus non-essentials – by even a small amount, you can decide how to spend this surplus on the nonessentials more wisely or how to begin saving it. Either way, you will want to start looking at ways to reduce b) – money out – and begin to feel more confident that you can live within your means.

After doing this audit on one of your first Money Diet days you can then return to it once a week, or once a fortnight, to check how much your monthly living costs have decreased.

I began to sketch my family's income and outgoings using the checklist above, and there were two surprises: I found it extremely satisfying to finally confront my deepest fears, and I also discovered that there's no reason why we couldn't live within our means if we were more careful.

The fact that we routinely managed to fail to do this was something I hoped to positively redress twice a week, while keeping an eye on our finances for the remaining five.

I live on my own and don't have children, so in theory I should be able to live comfortably off my salary of just over £2,000 a month as a shop manager, but I inevitably go overdrawn every month. I can't stand looking at my finances so this exercise was initially hard work, but once I sat down with a bank statement I felt quite organised. Some of it was a surprise – I didn't realise I was still paying for insurance on a washing machine that I no longer own!

I'm what you'd describe as "relaxed" about my finances – I never bother to go to comparison websites or change utility suppliers to get a better deal, but seeing on my audit that I pay £25 a month for my mobile phone made me wonder if I should change companies – I asked a friend and she only pays £18 a month for a fancier phone than mine, so I could save nearly £100 a year on that alone. It was interesting to see what I considered part of normal spending was actually nonessential, according to the audit. I need to look smart for work so I can justify buying new clothes regularly, but perhaps not quite as often as I do.

Vicky, 24

2 Set goals

Once you have those three magic figures – money in, money out and the figure that you need to cover your essentials each month – you can begin to set goals. Use the figures you've worked out as your guide as to where change is needed most.

Get specific about what you want to achieve. What do you really want from your 5:2 Money Diet days? To feel more in control emotionally? To start saving for a pension? To pay off your mortgage? To stop living in denial and feel less anxious about money? To save money for a particular treat or event? Or to just really get grips with the money and outgoings you have on a weekly and monthly basis?

Take a pen and paper and jot down your top five. Mine looked like this:

1) To feel better off: on average, my daily spending on myself and my family is around £40 a day. (To reach this figure, I took my monthly total from b) in Step 1, minus my fixed debits and standing orders, divided by four for a weekly sum, then seven to give me a daily spend). With two money-free days, I would save £80 a week – I want to visualise that £320 each month dropping into a high-savings account. I want to look forward to affording a meal out once a fortnight with my husband to share more time together (see 5:2 Your Relationship).

2) Feel happier: I want to rid myself of that general anxiety when I see our unfiled statements and bills breeding in the kitchen cupboard, and increase wellbeing by knowing we're in control of our finances.

3) Feel satisfied: I want a space to rest and reflect on how I consume for the rest of the week – be it screen-time, alcohol

or spending – my 5:2 Money Diet day will combine all three.

4) Feel more in control: I want to curb impulse-shopping and get to the root of why I give in to it.

5) Feel money efficient: I want to stay on top of my personal finances and know that I can live within my means.

This is an exercise you can sometimes return to on your Money Diet day because what you want to achieve may change as you continue with the 5:2 ratio, or you may want to aim for bigger, or smaller, goals.

Use your goals as incentives when the going gets tough. If you have that list handy, you're much more likely to stay enthusiastic and committed.

Vicky's top five goals:

1) To own my own flat.

2) To visit my friend in New Zealand.

3) To buy a new car.

4) To know how much money I have left by the end of the month, rather than hope for the best and cross fingers at the cash machine.

5) To feel that I am improving my situation rather than going up a down-escalator financially.

3 Restricted-Money Days

You've examined your financial situation, decided where savings could be made and drawn up a financial wish list. That's the planning over. Now you need to factor in something more active, a change to push you out of your familiar comfort zone and make you think and feel differently about the way you spend money. A happy side-effect of this jolt to your usual spending patterns twice a week is that your long-term habits will change too.

So challenge yourself to slashing your spending twice a week and have two restricted-money days (RMDs). If you're feeling really tough, go for a money-free day (MFD) as a one-off experience, or even once a week – no credit cards, no cash, no online spending. 'I have clients who would do anything rather than go a day without spending money,' says Simonne Gnessen, founder of Wise Monkey Financial Coaching and co-author of *Sheconomics*. 'So at first it's probably better to say, "OK, this is how much I've got to play with"' – go for the bare essentials rather than cutting out altogether. Or take a set amount of money but leave behind any credit and debit cards.

But if you do dare to go money free, you'll be surprised how liberating it can feel. 'Make sure you've got petrol in your car or a train ticket and something for lunch,' says Pine. 'At first it's quite a scary thing but you will get used to it.' Go to a gallery or a museum. Pick up a free newspaper. Go foraging, be imaginative. If you focus on what you can get for nothing rather than what you can spend, it's such an eye-opener.

If you want to work up to this one slowly, and you can trust yourself not to succumb to temptation, take your wallet or card with you for emergencies, if that makes you feel more reassured.

On your standard RMDs twice a week, simply cut down to a sum that feels realistic to you. 'You could try a maximum of £10 in cash and say that's it for today,' says Somerset Webb. 'The 5:2 food diet is incredibly simple and this should be too – don't complicate it, and stick to your ground rules.'

If you plan well, it doesn't have to be daunting or feel

uncomfortable. Rather like hunger pangs, the desire to spend money will pass. You'll feel stronger, more in control and satisfied on two counts: that the urge to spend can be resisted and that, bottom line, you've saved money.

Think of it as the 500-calorie fast as opposed to nil by mouth, it will still challenge and force you out of a comfort zone. But aim for nil by wallet either as a one-off experience and see how it makes you feel, a once-fortnightly or even monthly challenge. When you're not on your Money Diet, ignore it – it isn't how you live every day. Remind yourself that normal service can be resumed before you know it.

> *I normally spend around £10–£20 a day if I'm at work – this includes lunch in a café, a snack and a drink after work. If I see something I like in the shops during my lunch hour it could be much more – adding an extra £12 for a DVD or £50 for a jumper. The idea of not going out for lunch or having any treats, edible or otherwise, depresses me, but then so does my overdraft. If I had two money-free days I'd save £20–£40 a week and stay in the black. I think I equate being financially secure with being sensible, not very rock-and-roll, but in reality paying bank charges every month isn't great.*
>
> Joe, 30

Remember:

- *No* nonessentials.

- *No* shopping online.

- Be prepared. Ensure you are stocked up on essentials (keep an eye out for good deals) so that you are not caught without items such as milk, toothpaste, nappies, batteries, loo roll, which could ambush you on your no-/low-spending day.

On my first MFD, I decided to go hardcore and leave my wallet at home. I headed into central London with the children. What could possibly go wrong? My pre-loaded Oyster card got us all to South Kensington, where we strolled round the Victoria and Albert Museum and then sat on the steps eating sandwiches that I had made earlier that morning. Money wasn't an issue until we went back in and passed the museum gift shop. 'Can't we just have a look?' asked my middle one. I've always loved a museum gift shop, guiltily looking forward to the shopping nirvana of postcards, books and jewellery as much as seeing anything on display. 'Of course, but we can't buy anything.' Moans from my daughter, and secretly I completely agreed with her. 'It's important to be able to look and appreciate something, knowing you can't take it home and own it yourself,' I said, as much to myself as to her. 'Anyway, if there's something we really like in there,' I said, spotting a pair of earrings, 'we can always have a look online tomorrow.' Hopefully by the next day, this particular consumer pang would have passed.

I make sure that I combine one of my two Money Diet days with going to work – I take in sandwiches and cut out my mid-morning cappuccino, delighting in saving around £15 a day as a consequence. Even family Money Diet days are enjoyable, and not as difficult or extreme as I expected – a trip to the park, always taking lunch and water wherever I go, tuned in to anything I can get for free – with the help of websites like www.timeout.com/london/cheap-london. If you're outside London, www.dofreestuff.co.uk and www.visitbritain.com/en/Cheap-and-free-Britain/ are excellent sources of ideas.

'Your money-free day is a brilliant time to go wandering around the actual shops, as opposed to online,' says Merryn Somerset Webb. 'Once you've committed to not spending, it's a great freedom. You can say you'll come back knowing you won't really have the time. Or, if you do return, it will be because you've made a considered decision to make that purchase.'

I aimed for a zero spend for two days a week and the first one was hard. I took sandwiches but didn't bring enough and felt peckish around 3 p.m. I couldn't go to the choc dispenser and had to brave it out, eyeing my colleague and trying not to salivate as he munched his Maltesers. I forgot to take something to read too, so my commute was dreary. The second day was much better – my packed lunch was a veritable feast and I had plenty to last all afternoon. I also remembered to bring a section of the Sunday paper that I never get round to reading, for the journey to and from work, rather than buying a paper. I noticed that by not popping into the newsagent's at the station I also had to do without chewing gum and a bottle of water – saving £3. Next time I'll bring some from home.

I didn't dare to leave my wallet at home but I emptied it of cash to avoid temptation, just leaving my cash card for emergencies. I felt a bit tight during the whip-round for a colleague's birthday, so donated the next day. Some colleagues were going for a swift half after work, but I didn't join them. It wasn't a problem as I was combining a money-free day with an alcohol-free day, killing two birds with one stone.

I didn't enjoy the feeling of being deprived of my usual rituals of chocolate and newspapers during the first attempt – I'm not a pauper, so why should I live like one? – but the smug feeling of being prepared and saving money the second time round made up for it. I realised that I buy things to treat myself and make the working day more tolerable. Perhaps I need other ways to make myself feel better. '

James, 29

4 Cut your fixed costs

Don't assume that it's only disposable cash on your Money Diet days that you can reduce. Commit to reducing your fixed costs by 10 per cent – or a set amount that feels achievable for you.

Identify one standing order each week – internet provider, mobile phone, home insurance – and see if you could cut back. You may be paying extra on all sorts of monthly bills without realising it, and a simple check could shave off that wasted 10 per cent. Areas where you might be able to make savings include:

- Mobile phone insurance.

- Mobile phones and broadband: check the tariff is not set too high for your usage; check whether your phone is due for an upgrade and negotiate a SIM-only contract instead, which could be up to a quarter of the cost of your current monthly deal.

- Subscriptions to a film- or music-streaming site, like LOVEFiLM, Netflix or Spotify: monthly payments could be reduced or cut entirely if not used regularly.

- Travel or phone insurance on a credit card you don't require.

- A gym membership you don't need and could replace with exercising at home or in the park in half the time with the same health benefits and for free: see 5:2 Your Fitness.

- Home or car insurance: if it seems high, consider increasing the excess to decrease the annual premium.

Use price-comparison websites to help you make better decisions. Don't go to the same company for all your different insurances or loans. Saying that, could grouping your mobile, landline and broadband together save money? How does your energy provider or mobile phone company compare to other ones out there – look into what sort of savings you could make.

Start reading the financial pages of newspapers for introductory 0% interest rates on credit cards, and transfer any existing credit card balances onto the best.

If you're in debt, work on a strategy to pay it off during one of your Money Diet days. Talk to a free debt advice agency, or could you use the money you save on these two days to pay more than the minimum amount on your credit card bill each month? 'As an absolute rule, never make a minimum payment only on your credit cards,' advises Gnessen. 'Depending on the interest rates, it could take you around fifty years to pay it off. Always pay something more.'

Use the 'debt snowball', much loved by lifehackers. Pay off your smallest debt or credit card balance first, and then add the amount you were paying to service your first debt to the next. So if you were paying £50 on your first card and £100 on the second, when you pay off the first, you can increase the amount on the second to £150. It feels extremely gratifying to pick off one card then the next, and watch your debts decrease.

> *I found it satisfying thinking about ways I could save on each household bill; it became something of a challenge to shave off even a few pounds from every provider I had to pay. I switched my landline, mobile and broadband to one new provider and they gave me a big discount as a result of getting all three. I increased my excess payment on my house*

and car insurance, since I've never had to use them anyway. I also looked at the small print on my credit card and got rid of my travel insurance, which I never knew was there. Overall saving for half an hour's work? £75 a month.

Louisa, 35

I started lift-sharing to get to work by finding someone who does practically the same commute as me (www.liftshare.com). We alternate weeks driving so one of us can relax and read the paper. We don't feel the need to make polite conversation; mostly we listen to the radio and it has become an easy way to save money. The added bonus is that I'm never late now – curiously, I find it easier to be on time for my lift than I do to get to work on time by myself. Money-wise, I used to fill up once a week for around £60, now that's down to once a fortnight.

Sam, 34

As you'll discover from your money audit, one of your biggest outgoings is food shopping. With food prices increasing by 3 per cent a year and wages by only 1 per cent, this is an area where you ought to focus your 5:2 Money Diet.

Always be prepared before you buy online or at the supermarket. Here are some money-saving tips:

- Before you go shopping, check what you already have in stock and think how you might use it next week.

- Vet expiry dates: make sure you use food you've already bought in good time and that new purchases have as long a shelf life as possible.

- Look at your calendar to check what days you're out, and therefore how many meals you will need to prepare that week.

- Remember your bags – most supermarkets now charge you for extra ones; on the other hand, some reward you with points for bringing your own.

- Check websites like www.mysupermarket.com to track and stock up on savvy buys.

- Shop for extras in the evenings when many supermarkets will start discounting fresh produce.

- For smaller shops, always avoid a trolley. A basket will demand that you focus on essential rather than nonessential buys.

- Stock up on store-cupboard items that are on special offer.

5 Confront your money demons

If there's one process you should ensure you undergo twice a week, it's managing your financial affairs and responsibilities. How often do you look at your account? Do you open and file bills and bank statements as soon as you receive them? Do you postpone tasks like filling in your tax return?

Commit a small amount of time on your two designated days – no more than fifteen minutes – during which you engage with one specific aspect of your personal finances. One segment of time could be devoted to checking your account online, to re-indexing all your papers or to checking that all your bills are up-to-date and on the lowest possible tariff. Use that small window to organise your paperwork. If there's a big pile in the corner that you don't want to look at, commit to five minutes at first and then build to ten, then come back on your second day. Much easier to tell yourself 'I'm going to do this task for five minutes,' rather than 'I'm going to do this whole task brilliantly right now'.

Focus on how many different accounts you have yourself or jointly with your partner, including mortgage, savings, junior ISAs, investments, making sure that your money is in the most productive places, balancing the accessibility you need against the higher interest rates available for accounts where withdrawing money might incur penalties.

Facing up to our money fears isn't only about confronting current debts, it's about planning and being realistic about your savings for the future too. It's useful to have a figure in mind so you can think about the type of retirement you envisage or perhaps a move or change in lifestyle in the near future. Gnessen suggests that while you have all your statements to hand that you ask yourself 'How much am I worth?' 'If you were to cash in everything – pensions, savings, and pay off your mortgage – what are you left with? Your aim is for that amount to grow. By the time you stop working, by how much would you need to see it build for you to have a comfortable amount to live on?' You could consider increasing your pension contributions and savings, or more actively engaging with your mortgage.

Think about your current mortgage deal – when does it come to an end? Could you get a better deal by switching? If you have an interest-only mortgage, could you afford to switch to repayment? Mortgages are like credit cards: you should always aim to pay off more than the monthly minimum fee if you can do so, or save into a separate account to 'over-pay' within your limit at the end of each year.

Find out about employer offers that you may not know about – supermarket vouchers, share option schemes, opportunities to increase your pension and childcare vouchers.

> *The game-changer for me on my second MFD was facing up to what scared me most. My husband and I are too similar, often avoiding looking at bank statements or bills, willing the other one to take control, but I or he never will. Yet now, the simple commitment of looking at our account online once a week has taken away so much anxiety. And we've discovered that we're not as badly off as we assumed. We've got a list of all the days our standing orders debit, so we know when we can spend money. We're so much happier, we pay less in charges, spend almost nothing twice a week, and we're better off by around £300 a month.*
> Lottie, 36

I admit I was extremely resistant to this step. I'm much happier taking extreme action in the moment – as in spending nothing all day. But sitting down with paperwork makes me feel resentful, fearful and slightly overwhelmed. Filing my bills and checking online statements was the very last task I wanted to sit down to on a Monday evening – my first MFD – and the only one I kept putting off in the 5:2 life areas. I found it much easier when I timed myself – I gave myself twenty-five minutes (see the Pomodoro technique on p.149 in 5:2 Your Productivity) to see how far I could get and it instantly removed the dread of feeling that it would eat away my evening.

6 Seven ways to help cut your spending

1) The more aware you are of your bank balance, what's coming in when and what's just gone out, the more controlled you'll be about your spending overall. A good tip from Gnessen: change your homepage on your

computer to show your bank's website page, which will remind you to check your balance every few days on one of your RMDs. Like a Post-it note on your front door, you can't ignore it.

2) Avoid online shopping websites on your Money Diet days and, the next day, if you do browse, give yourself a forty-eight-hour cooling-off period. If you see something you're desperate to buy, consign it to your wish list. When you revisit, ask a friend or partner to take a look. They're more likely to be objective than you.

3) Get the Save It! app. 'This is fantastic – you can use it on your MFD and for everything you don't buy that you would normally have reached for; scan it in and see how much you've saved at the end of those two days. Transfer that money from your current account into an MFD savings account and you can see immediate progress,' says Somerset Webb.

4) Think about money in a different way by taking a leaf out of the recent 'frugality hackers' movement, focused around websites including www.beingfrugal.net and www.getrichslowly.org, and in the UK, www.frugalfamily.co.uk. These sites encourage a different mindset: to feel content living within your means, as opposed to saving now in the hope of spending more later.

5) *Get on your bike!* Think about your transport and where you could cut costs – why not gain green points for 5:2 Your Environment and cycle? Or buy a fold-up bike and combine with a train ride, if you commute? You can save up to 42 per cent on any bike with the government's Cycle to Work tax exemption initiative. See www.cyclescheme.co.uk,

www.bike2workscheme.co.uk, or www.cycle2work.info to find out how to sign up.

> *I was frustratingly standing on a packed – and delayed – Tube last summer trying to get to work thinking, "Why do I pay so much money for such a poor service? There must surely be an easier, cheaper way." A colleague at work recommended I get a fold-up bike through my company's Cycle to Work scheme. It was a light-bulb moment. The following week I bought one for £500 (saving over £200, and paying for it in monthly instalments) and haven't looked back. I actually get to work ten minutes quicker by bike and save approximately £88 a week on my commute (before it was a ten-minute bus ride and then thirty minutes by Tube), so the bike paid for itself after just six months. Now I put the monthly £88 saving directly into a cash ISA which will pay for a skiing holiday I've planned for next March. I don't include the money I save by using the bike at weekends, I just put that in my mental Smug Bank. So what's not to like? I save over a £1,000 a year and get fit in the process. I don't understand why everyone with a short enough commute doesn't do the same.*
>
> Robert, 44

6) Never go to a supermarket to do your big shop if you can possibly help it, advises Somerset Webb. 'Always do a weekly grocery shop online and even then stick to a strict list.' You can then top up on essential fresh produce or anything more unusual in person, but don't be tempted by deals for things you don't need or won't use. Never do any food shop, online or otherwise, on an empty stomach.

7) Focus on what you can earn on your Money Diet days, not what you can spend. 'Don't just think, "How much money

can I save?"' says Pine, 'but rather, "How much money can I make?"' What can you sell on eBay? Collect all the small change from under the bed, on your desk, behind the radio and convert at the supermarket.

As part of changing my overall attitude to money, the screensaver has really worked for me. The more I check my current account, the less I splurge. The opposite is equally true – the more in the dark I am about my financial situation, the easier I find it to be irresponsible and spend thoughtlessly. Which is why it's so important for me to stay in the loop. I only spend less when I'm really engaged and involved in where all my money is going.

    Kate, 30

I don't do online banking ever since I was the victim of internet fraud, so checking my balance involves ringing up or going to the cash machine. One reason I never knew how much I had was because I always had to look up the number for the bank – a hassle. Now I've added it to my mobile phone contacts, it's much easier.

    Jane, 29

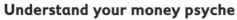

7 Understand your money psyche

Our relationship to money is complex: so much so that it is hard to think of another commodity in our culture that stirs up more feeling. Accept that our attitude towards money is rarely rational and work with that reality. Understanding why this should be so requires some self-reflection.

Along with the record you're keeping of what you spend, as outlined in Step 1, a great way of examining your attitudes to money is to write down your feelings in any situation where money crops up – spending it, checking it or talking about it – on two days of each week. Look at your notes at the end of these days: are there any particular catalysts, events or even people that bring about certain emotions?

> After two weeks of keeping a diary of my feelings around money, I began to see patterns, how certain emotions pop up again and again, mainly guilt and regret. I share my bank account with my boyfriend and I always feel bad if I buy something that isn't for both of us – I noticed at least two notes I'd made after I bought some books and some trainers. "I feel guilty but at least they're not too frivolous. Maybe I just won't tell him for a while and hope he doesn't notice in our account."
>
> I notice that I've made fewer notes about what I buy than the conversations I have, particularly with my mother, about money and why this could be significant. In one note I've written "money = anxiety". I freelance and whenever I try to reassure her by saying I've just got more work, she says, "But what will you do after that, if and when the work runs out?" I have a stronger sense of why I always associate money with worry.
>
> Jen, 32

Thinking about your money and your childhood is another powerful way to work out how your emotions shape and define your spending habits.

Our parents' financial attitudes can reveal so much about our own responses and particularly what money symbolises in our own life – control, power, security, love etc. To what extent are we repeating family patterns, and are we even aware of it? The following exercise will help you find out.

Think about the following questions or discuss them if you're doing the exercise with a friend, relation or partner.

- What was your mother's attitude to money? And your father's?

- Did they share their finances?

- Who earned more – your mother or father? Did this influence who made the big financial decisions?

- Who had more control generally over decision-making in your family – over holidays, schooling, where you lived? To what extent was this linked, if at all, to who controlled the finances?

> *My father lives up to the reputation of the Yorkshireman who is very careful with money. This has generally made me responsible when it comes to spending on a daily basis. However, I also find myself splurging on things he would never buy if he didn't have the ready cash, whereas my attitude is to think that I'll get paid next week and it will most likely be OK: needless to say, I'm not a big fan of checking my bank balance at that point in the month. Being more aware of how much I have to spend week-by-week has definitely helped to curb these impulse purchases.*
>
> Sarah, 30

> *Both my parents were very casual about money. My dad earned a good salary as a doctor but he paid emergency tax for years because he never examined his pay slips. Bills were in a huge pile in the study and my mum was too bohemian to stress about the cost of living. I too shared their view until I moved to London and had a low-paid job. I was shocked out of my bubble and had to start budgeting for things.*
>
> Abi, 33

My dad was very generous with money and always liked to give big dinner parties, spending lots on the very best food and drinks. My mum winced at his attitude and was in control of the family budget for the rest of the week. I have grown up wanting to be careful with money but find some economising a bore. I feel a mixture of awe and contempt for my sister-in-law who knows the price of every item in Sainsbury's and goes to different supermarkets for different groceries to save money.

Jenny, 39

Now sit down with a pen and paper, and reflect on the following statements – to what extent do you agree/disagree? Explain for each comment. If relevant, try to involve your partner too.

- I love the idea of being rich
- Money doesn't make you happy
- I wish I earned more money
- I'm impressed when someone tells me how wealthy they are
- I feel someone hasn't succeeded if they don't make much money
- There is never enough money in my life
- If I'm feeling down, I deserve to cheer myself up shopping
- If I've done well at work, I deserve to reward myself shopping

Take two or three minutes to think about or discuss these statements. Examining, reflecting on and discussing these assumptions will help you to shed light on your beliefs and attitudes to money, how deep-rooted they are and where they come from.

If you're in a relationship, it's a good opportunity to think about how you both deal with money as a couple – where does conflict arise? Where do attitudes and emotions differ most – is one of you a spender and one a hoarder?

Use the reflective listening tool in 5:2 Your Relationship (p.192) to explore these issues further. Let your partner talk for five minutes uninterrupted about anything on his or her mind that's money-related while you listen and repeat back the main points, reflecting their thoughts and feelings in an empathetic way. Discussing money can often trigger powerful irrational responses, so this is a great way of understanding your partner's point of view, as well as feeling understood yourself, in a safe and neutral context.

Remember, resolving money differences isn't easy; it's an eternal conflict because money represents pleasure on the one hand and security on the other – squaring wants and needs is challenging enough alone, but even more difficult within a couple.

How to resist

When the impulse to buy strikes, here are some techniques to help you battle the urge:

- Feel that desire to buy and say, 'No, I can come back and buy it tomorrow or next week.' Or simply say, 'I can do without this.' Rather than seeing it as a deprivation, view it as a way of standing back, being aware of how you're being manipulated.

- Have pre-set questions – in the back of your mind or written down – that require a 'yes' answer before you can buy. 'Do I really need this?', 'Do I really want it?', 'Do I have money in my account to cover it?'

- Visualise your goals in Step 2 when you feel an impulse taking over. 'If it's the deposit for a mortgage, picture a house and how much you want it,' says Gnessen. What you're trying to do is introduce something – an idea or picture – that interrupts the stimulus response dynamic, creating a pause between wanting something and actually buying it.

- Think about carrying other reminders in your wallet to break the impulse. 'I made one client a credit-card-sized laminate with two numbers on – one was her net worth and the other were her credit card debts. Whenever she reached for her credit card, she would see it,' says Gnessen.

My rationale when an impulsive urge takes over is "How did I feel five minutes ago before I spotted this item? My life was content and replete before I knew it existed, and will be so again if I can walk away now." Ten minutes later, I'll remind myself, "See, you feel as happy now as if you'd bought that thing, probably more so because you're slightly better off." I feel good afterwards and that memory makes it easier to achieve each time. This mantra has saved me many hundreds of pounds over the last year alone.
    Philippa, 35

I remind myself of the pain of having to return an item bought online if it doesn't fit – queuing at the Post Office, filling out that tedious form. So much easier not to have it at all!
    Tessa, 31

I love reading the books on prize shortlists, but it is a costly habit. I order them at the library instead now – yes, you

have to wait for them, but it only costs seventy pence a book instead of at least a tenner.
Eleanor, 54

COMMON QUESTIONS

Why do I need to do this?

If money worries keep you awake at night or you find it increasingly daunting to face up to your overdraft or credit card debts, these 5:2 Money Diet steps will help you take practical steps to overcome these feelings. Or perhaps you turn to shopping when you're down to cheer yourself up, or do it when you're happy to maintain that feeling, and instead want to plan your purchases more carefully so that they are not dictated by your mood.

Which two days should I choose?

Choose non-consecutive days as RMDs so that you can remind yourself that a no-spending day may feel tough today but ends tomorrow. For maximum saving, build up to one MFD a week, ultimately at the weekend when you're likely to spend the most. If this feels too brutal, stick to two weekdays when you're busier at work or home and less likely to shop.

Which other 5:2 life areas combine well with my Money Diet?

 Your 5:2 **Screen Life** Diet is an ideal partner to the 5:2 **Money** Diet – a digital detox takes away one major source of temptation: online shopping. Combine with your 5:2

 Drink Diet too – though not on the same days – think of the money you'll save on that bottle of wine, and if you're on the 5:2 diet as well, you're cutting calories and saving even more money on food.

FINANCE FACTS

- Money anxieties can temporarily lower your intelligence, according to research. In IQ tests, scientists found that those with money worries performed much worse – as many as thirteen points fewer – than those with more money.

- Don't go shopping under a cloud – a survey published in *Psychology and Marketing* journal found that if you are in a bad mood you are more likely to buy something to cheer yourself up.

- What you have in your purse affects whether you spend it. Having £10 in change makes you a lot more likely to spend it than a £10 note, according to a study in the *Journal of Consumer Research*. The researchers argue that larger notes are also treated as less flexible than smaller ones, which is why people are reluctant to spend them.

- If you feel down, you're more likely to spend more, says a study published in the journal *Psychological Science*. After participants watched a sad video, designed to trigger unhappy emotions, they offered to pay nearly four times as much money to buy a water bottle than a group that watched an emotionally neutral clip.

5:2

YOUR PRODUCTIVITY

LIFE BEFORE MY 5:2 PRODUCTIVITY FIX

It's midday, and I am staring at one solitary paragraph marooned on my screen. I should have stockpiled a thousand words by now, crowded out that blank expanse with dense sentences, well-ordered paragraphs, glorious black print signifying a morning's achievement. Somehow I haven't. More minutes pass and panic flutters.

I'm not in the zone, I tell myself, as if I have no choice in the matter. I am weak-willed, overtaken by the slightest impulse or excuse to waste yet another five minutes 'researching' on Wikipedia, online newspapers, magazines and gossip sites. I don't *really* want to read about the state of Pippa Middleton's bottom, or why Simon Cowell welcomes fatherhood, but somehow I get drawn in.

I could go offline altogether, as many writers recommend, but I'm not sure how much that would help. I'd only end up emptying the dishwasher, cleaning that cobweb in the hallway, paying the TV licence or reading a book. Anything but the task in hand. I enjoy writing but when it's an urgent priority, I'll seek out any distraction.

Yet procrastination experts would say it isn't laziness, or even a weakness for vapid celebrity stories (although I suspect the latter doesn't help) but a deliberate avoidance strategy. There's a reason I'm resisting the task in hand, they'd conclude: it's due to a fear of truly engaging, masking yet deeper fears of failure or rejection. I'm not convinced. I don't feel there's any unconscious ambivalence; it feels more like a shift in mood and energy that is somehow beyond my control.

For a short time I can feel highly motivated, able to burn through the most daunting of tasks and then, without warning, that resolve evaporates and online distractions beckon. That's because, according to productivity experts, our energy levels fluctuate throughout the day. I should focus on working in short bursts and view my willpower in a different way.

My approach to any work assignment or project has always been to try and carve out long days where I can sit in a room 'until the task is done', not daring to walk away, rest or do something different, for fear inspiration will strike at any moment and I may miss my chance. My golden period of productivity rarely lasts more than three hours, so why can't I just work for that amount of time and relax for the rest, rather than spending many hours in a muddled combination of the two?

While completing a particularly long work project, I decided to stay with my mother-in-law in Cornwall, free from all distractions. Long, luxurious stretches of time yawned before me as I sat in her small study, knowing I could write until dawn if I wished. Surely working would be easier without the limitations of office hours, school pick-ups, meal times and domestic routine? Yet all that silence, space and freedom, locked away for ten-hour days, made the task that lay before me seem all the more elusive. I'm not sure I was any more productive than I would have been working at home, where I have to write more quickly, knowing I might be ambushed at any moment by a waking baby.

This would come as no surprise to productivity expert and CEO of the Energy Project Tony Schwarz, who believes creating limitations actually helps our willpower and efficiency. Knowing we've only got a set time to complete a task (Schwarz believes ninety minutes is the optimum), followed by a period of renewal, is the best way to work. It's the recovery time, he believes, that can allow for the most creativity – running, walking, day-dreaming even – before you get back to those focused stints.

A sprinter sustains his impressive speed, he suggests, because there's a finishing line he can see. Not unlike 5:2 itself – it means creating restrictions that can allow us to thrive, i.e. have two days of short but intense bursts of productivity with a tangible end within our grasp.

MAKING THE 5:2 CONNECTION

I already knew from my research into high intensity interval training (HIIT), (see 5:2 Your Fitness), that the body responds well to timed high-intensity challenges, alternating strenuous effort with short recovery times.

In my first taste of HIIT with personal trainer Steve Mellor, I completed a brief but punishing round of exercises applying the Tabata principle of twenty seconds on and ten seconds off for four minutes of effort. It was challenging – partly because I had a personal trainer standing over me and pushing me to my limit – but it was all over within twenty minutes, including a warm-up and cool-down. I was left feeling a little shaky, but also alert and invigorated – not a word I've often, if ever, used when it comes to me and exercise. I carried on feeling 'invigorated' for the rest of the morning, so much so that I decided, while still in this rare state, to apply the technique to my work. I focused intensely for thirty minutes on a piece of writing, then rested for ten, tried it again three times and then gave myself a longer recovery time. Somehow, it worked. I powered through a piece of work that would normally have taken me a long and languid afternoon. All the better, it was a task I had been avoiding.

What seemed to activate me was moving swiftly from intense exercise to an equally intense work mode, transferring all the energy from one arena to another quite different one, and resting in between.

I approached Fergus O'Connell, CEO, project manager and author of *The Power of Doing Less*, who could immediately see the benefits of applying 5:2 to work productivity. 'It's a very nonthreatening idea of making behavioural changes, to be able to say, "I'll try this on a Tuesday or Thursday and then regroup and get my courage back."'

Graham Allcott, founder of Think Productive and author of *How to Be a Productivity Ninja*, can also see the promise. 'It's a fascinating area because 5:2 is all about constraints and constraints can be very productive.'

THE 5:2 PRODUCTIVITY FIX; aims and benefits

- A moderate way to boost productivity twice a week, increasing efficiency every day.

- Enjoyable exercises that you can return to as your goals and challenges change, as well as techniques that can become part of your daily 5:2 plan.

- Work harder but in shorter bursts. Relax more, savour your renewal and recovery time at the weekends.

- Learn to set boundaries and to relax as 'productively' as you work: remember that productivity doesn't relate only to work – if you spend two days on holiday but fail to switch off, it hasn't been a 'productive' break.

- Making small changes, for example clearing your inbox to zero, will have an impact on your whole week, make you feel more in control and therefore more motivated.

- Feel more assertive; discover how to say 'no' nicely without fear of criticism or rejection.

- Combine your fitness and work interval training for the ultimate productivity boost.

GETTING STARTED ON THE 5:2 PRODUCTIVITY FIX

These steps outline exercises and reflections to help you make small changes on your two productivity days, and also invite you to think about the 5:2 ratio in different ways – as a model for making the most of your 'two-day' weekend, as well as a daily ratio: two hours of doing something slightly different within a typical seven-hour working day. Mix and match these thoughts and ideas to help you think about the importance of self-imposed constraints – be they daily or weekly – and why setting your own realistic 'interval times' is the cornerstone of productivity.

SEVEN STEPS TO MAKE THE 5:2 PRODUCTIVITY FIX WORK FOR YOU

1 Set to zero

Use two hours of your 5:2 Productivity Fix to clean up, catch up and take stock. 'If you've only got two days each week to stay productive, this is the most important thing you can do,' says productivity guru David Allen and bestselling author of *Getting Things Done.*

'That first day should be given to cleaning up your backlog, lifting your head above the fray,' says Allen. It's what he calls 'getting current' and 'knowing your inventory'. Answering telephone messages and clearing your inbox of emails as far as possible will give you an overview of your most pressing demands and projects. Don't even think about priorities or goals until you've taken this simple and satisfying step.

There's no better place to start than with your email: decluttering your inbox is guaranteed to make you feel more productive. Email overflow can feel like a physical weight representing the eternal queue of unmet requests and demands in every area of your life. So strip it away.

As author Oliver Burkeman writes in *Help!: How to Become Slightly Happier and Get a Bit More Done*, 'There's something weirdly addictive about the blankness of an empty inbox which makes you want to keep it that way.'

It will also give you a fair idea of what really needs to be done, and what doesn't. The payoff? How can you not start each day with a Zen-like calm thanks to an inbox that is more a tranquil temple than a crowded shopping mall?

Here's how:

1) Think of your inbox as your hallway – no one wants to wade knee-high through letters and parcels to reach the front door each morning. Nor should you be scrolling down endless pieces of mail every morning.

2) Since this could be the first time you've pruned your inbox, don't expect to be able to tackle it all at once. Accept that the first two attempts may take you a while. Begin by creating a separate folder called 'archive', if you haven't already set one up, and move *everything* from your inbox into here. Take a moment to glory in that pristine inbox you have now created.

3) Set aside twenty-five minutes and time yourself (see the Pomodoro technique in Step 7) or Tabata your inbox in longer chunks (also Step 7). With each mail in your 'archive', simply delete, unsubscribe, file by project, or label it as in need of a response later – it might be easier to sort by name or subject as you work through them. Take a five- or ten-minute break and then set the timer again. Keep a list and note down any outstanding tasks that crop up during your ruthless pruning.

4) You must repeat this process once, ideally twice, a week on your productivity days to maintain the regular high of email nirvana. Once your inbox is clear, you'll also find less excuse, and incentive, to continually click onto it as a diversion activity.

5) Many productivity experts, from Merlin Mann on www.43folders.com to David Allen, recommend inbox-

emptiness as a daily goal. This is probably a demand too far for the 5:2 ratio; in fact part of this step is simply accepting that a blank inbox is a transient joy. Demands will mount up and clutter will accumulate, and you don't have to control this influx all the time. It might be better to acknowledge it and let it be, knowing that you'll be able to dedicate time to sort through it again soon. (See mindfulness meditations in 5:2 Your Worry, p.219). Otherwise the white zero challenge becomes yet another demand that weighs on you. So recognise that tasks can never be fully done: this is one you can return to once or twice a week. The rest of the time, focus on other things.

6) Here's a good shortcut from Allcott: 'Anything older than say, three months, move to a folder called "email death row". Then put an entry in your calendar for four to six weeks' time saying "Did I need anything that was in 'email death row'?" From there, you can review whether you need to spend any more time on that stuff – but it's more responsible than just deleting immediately.'

I am a technophobe and have emails in my inbox going back to 2006. I always read or delete new emails but didn't archive or put them into folders as I didn't know how. I bit the bullet and asked my partner how to and have got as far as the first ten pages, which goes back to July this year – all sorted into different folders: utilities, personal, work, and so on. It feels very unlike me. I get a little thrill when I get a new email and know where to tidy it away to.

Yvonne, 41

The notion of sorting out my inbox made me feel tired and that life was too short, but I gave it a go and discovered it has its merits. Previously, I would have to do a mental high jump over the spam, newsletters and Facebook notifications that I should have deleted but hadn't, to search for the interesting new emails. For the first couple of days it was clearer, less taxing and I'm also not distracted by irrelevant updates. It's building up again now though so, dreary as it is, I suppose I'll have to do it regularly.
    Jim, 53

Thinking outside the inbox

'I make a habit of clearing out my email inbox every morning before I start work; for me it's like making a coffee before I get on with the tasks of the day. I find it very cathartic – there's nothing worse than seeing 300 mails in your box first thing, as it immediately swamps you with Things I Must Do and sets you off in a state of panic. In reality, there's probably only ten or so emails that I actually have to action or even reply to. The rest I view as just unwelcome distractions. Once practised, it takes just ten minutes to clear out your inbox and it means you begin the day with a clean slate. It's the only way I can start to be creative, knowing I don't have a pile of emails hanging over me.

    'First of all I trawl through all the junk mails and delete immediately, without reading them, then I dump all emails from people whose names I don't recognise. I figure if it's important, they can always send another message. Then I look at the emails from people I do know and either reply straight away (the best option) or save to my "Action" folder, which means I'll reply by the end of the day or during one of my more unproductive moments, but never at weekends or after 6 p.m.

'Emails that I may need to action/reply to/reference go into my "Archive" folder. All other emails are superflous and must be deleted immediately. I also make sure my email alert is off so I don't get distracted during the day unnecessarily replying to emails. So, by around 9.30 a.m. I am ready to work. I will only look at my inbox again at 5 p.m. and then spend another ten minutes replying, deleting or archiving as before; this means my inbox in the morning will be an easily manageable fifty or so. For me, really, it's all about thinking outside the inbox!'

Jenny, 36

2 Priority audit

Often we can feel as if time is running out, that the volume of tasks that faces us is ever greater. Conventional time-management techniques offer advice on getting through the onslaught of work in a more efficient way, essentially teaching us how to cram more in to each day. Maybe we should be looking at it in a different way, accepting that much of what faces us will fall off a to-do list, and asking, 'Does that really matter?' This way of thinking can be empowering, says author Fergus O'Connell, especially if it helps us to make choices. 'Lots of stuff won't get done and we need to accept that. We can just let that happen or decide proactively what things we won't do. The more we decide, the more we'll live the life we want to live.' O'Connell's approach is to focus our productivity on the tasks that really matter, and discard the rest. What you need to work out is what really matters, and what's top of your daily to-do list should reflect these primary needs in some way.

Sit down with a pen and paper, set a timer for ten minutes, and think about your bucket list – the things you'd most like to spend your time doing if you suddenly found out you had less than a year to live. What matters most to you? Being more creative? Writing that novel? Giving up work altogether, spending time with your family, or starting a family? Going travelling? When the timer goes, reflect on this list. Are there any patterns here – wanting to be more ambitious, or change your life radically?

Here is the 'One-year-to-live' list of Karen, 32:

- Travel to somewhere exotic, e.g. Borneo.

- Build one-to-one relationships with my children and take time to do things with them individually.

- Teach myself to touch-type.

- Improve my piano-playing and play regularly.

- Tackle doing up our house instead of avoiding the work.

- Think about moving overseas for a year, e.g. New Zealand.

- Go and see live music regularly and learn to download music from the web.

- Be more proactive with work instead of waiting for it to come to me.

Now streamline your list, pruning it down to the big three – what small actions today could lead you to achieve or explore each of these as possibilities or even certainties? Bear them in mind when you do this next exercise: they should be at the top.

Set your timer again for a further ten minutes and think about your daily to-do list, your priorities for that day or week, and to what extent they aid or support the goals in your first list.

Karen's daily to-do list:

- Finish off newsletter for the PTA.
- Call my editor/boss/potential client back – i.e. an enquiry that could mean money.
- Make cupcakes for my daughter's year group home-bake.
- Try to reduce home insurance annual cost, which seems too high.
- Respond to a backlog of emails.
- Book appointment for haircut.
- Book appointment for dentist.
- Take books back to the library.

Reflect on these two lists and the links between them. Buried in the mundane slurry of daily demands, there should be connections revealing how you really want to spend your time – one should be in service to the other.

Karen's most crucial aims:

- To spend more time with her children on a one-to-one basis.

- To be more proactive with work.

- To do up the house.

My weekly list contained things that overlapped with my bucket list if I tweaked them. I could bake the cupcakes with my 3-year-old instead of doing them much more quickly in the evening. She would love it and I would feel I had had "quality time" with her.

When replying to emails I now try to suggest ideas to create more work rather than just respond to others.

I feel stymied about doing up the house because we don't have the money to do it, but that will be solved if more income comes in from my efforts.

Karen, 32

It's worth coming back to these two lists on your productivity days to reflect to what extent your everyday tasks match your overarching aims and priorities – at least half of your daily priorities should feed in and be devoted to your first list. If not, think of streamlining your daily to-do list using techniques suggested here.

For example, Fergus O'Connell is ruthless about making sure his daily activities – what he decides to do or to ignore – serve his bigger interests. If an email is a potential distraction from his greater aim, he'll ignore it. His strategy is ruthless, he admits, which is why he can combine two careers and not feel overwhelmed.

O'Connell manages his own business and is also a novelist. 'I see it as two full-time jobs but I manage to do both of them in around forty-five hours a week. I probably spend more time with my children than they'd like – I'm a family man. I also enjoy cooking and gardening. My forty-five hours is massively productive. If I was doing seventy to eighty hours, I know I wouldn't be. I never slog on for the sake of it, it's never worth it.'

His secret is asking only two questions before he initiates any task: 'Will this improve my business?' and 'Will this enable me to spend more time writing my books?' If it's a 'no', he'll move on. He calls it knowing the 'right stuff'. Get used to only doing what's really important on any list, deciding what's the 'right stuff'. 'Continually question what the right stuff is and stick to it,' he says.

'I prioritise existing customers and new business – sales enquiries. I could have fifteen emails and if they don't fall into either of those categories, I won't look at them on the day I'm writing. It means there's no dithering. If it doesn't match up with these incredibly important priorities, it won't get my focus.'

3 Just say no

In order to eliminate the incidental activity that makes demands on your time and holds you back from your ultimate goals, you need to learn to say no. O'Connell says, 'Paradoxically, not doing something requires work. That work comes from making things disappear.'

Saying no nicely is a skill that can only be acquired through practice and steely resolve. To a certain degree, we're all people-pleasers.

So an essential task for your productivity days is to say no at least once a day, hopefully dropping in this two-letter word two or three times by week three or four.

Sit down with a pen and paper and make a list of five ways to say no nicely – think of five tasks you were asked to do in the last two days that you didn't really want to do because you didn't feel they were worthwhile but, out of politeness, you did anyway. You can refer to your second list in Step 2 and think about which ones you wish you'd said no to. It doesn't matter how trivial or significant the demand is – from your partner asking you to empty the bins to a colleague requesting you take on an extra piece of work.

Here is the list of five things that Joanna, 40, wishes she'd said no to:

1) Going to a book group organised by a friend, which I don't enjoy. I just felt obliged because she was counting on me but inside I felt put upon. I don't like book groups because I don't like the 'lively' debate about them – I don't enjoy arguing!

2) Letting my daughter take toys to the park, which inevitably get lost and have to be searched for. I felt weak because she wears me down into agreeing even after I have said no.

3) Having pork chops for tea when I didn't feel like them, just because my partner suggested them. I felt like I was sacrificing my needs for the sake of avoiding conflict.

4) Staying up later than I wanted and drinking too much at a dinner party we held because I felt I couldn't ask people to go. I felt other people's opinion of me was more important than what I wanted.

5) Agreeing to a poorly paid work assignment because I didn't feel strong enough to negotiate and having to work far more than I had anticipated. It made me feel like I was being taken for granted and that I was too weak to get what I deserved.

Keeping a journal of when you successfully managed to say no just once on your productivity days will help you see how you can build on those skills. How did it make you feel? Gradually start saying no more frequently. Be conscious throughout that day that you're going to choose what you want and don't want to do; that you have a choice and you're going to follow the list that you made in Step 2.

> I'm a production manager for a film company and, in my office, I'm seen as super-efficient; in fact it's a running joke how organised I am. But it also means colleagues end up asking me to do extra stuff, flattering me by saying, "Come on, you're so organised, you'll get it done more quickly." Over the years I've had to learn how to say no and the trick is to be direct, don't give them wiggle room by saying, "I'll see, let's talk about it again tomorrow." A boomerang request will just come back harder than before. Start with an apology, "I'm sorry but ..." and then a really friendly but firm "No." Let them know your boundaries early on and stick to them.
> Michael, 45

> My daughter is the queen of pester-power: she ignores me saying no until I finally say yes. I have now taken to saying, "You don't need to ask again because you already know the answer," and repeat ad infinitum. She objected, naturally, but is now resigned to it. It has been helpful for our relationship because I often give in to her to avoid a meltdown but she can't hold me to ransom with it now. It reminded us both that I am the boss and she needs to accept that.
> Charlotte, 44

> I was asked if I would accept a one-off fee rather than a daily rate for a project I was involved in. I was put on the

spot on the telephone and would normally have agreed and then regretted it, but I managed to explain why the daily rate works better for me. My boss went away to examine the budget again, which made me feel nervous – had I just shot myself in the foot? But then I felt empowered when she came back with a fee that worked for both of us. I normally bend over backwards to accommodate other people so this was new and nerve-wracking but ultimately rewarding. I think perhaps it's good for our working relationship – she's less likely to try that again.
  Tony, 33

'This is a simple challenge but many people can find it difficult to get that victory, big or small', says O'Connell. 'If at first you don't succeed, do an action replay to see where you gave up, where you could build on that attempt next time.'

4 Slay your dragons

We all know those tasks that we least want to do. The ones that provoke the sense of telltale dread are invariably the ones that require most brainpower and effort. If you're resisting them, there's a reason, and you need to ask yourself why and then decide on the best time to tackle them. It's important to distinguish between the demands we would like to say 'no' to more because they lead us away from the goals of our bigger picture (see Step 2), and the tasks that feel daunting because they require our greatest energy and input, and can often be the most worthwhile. Often they're the very ones that lead us to our 'bigger picture' – in my case, hitting a writing deadline to finish a book. In my friend's case, it was completing very complex and time-consuming architectural plans to submit to the council so she could get on with building her dream home.

Stephen Covey, author of the bestseller *The 7 Habits of Highly Effective People*, famously describes these 'big tasks' as the rocks in our life, the heavy ones that must fit in the jar first before we pour the smaller demands – the pebbles and gravel – into the crevices and cracks around these giant boulders.

Similarly Brian Tracy's book *Eat That Frog* is based on the old saying 'If the first thing you do when you wake up in the morning is eat a frog, nothing worse can happen to you that day.' 'Eating a frog' should be at the top of your to-do list, he says, otherwise it will sit there draining your energy and making you feel guilty. Bolt back that slimy creature, he promises, and you'll overflow with energy and momentum for the rest of the day. It's very true that just the act of getting through something daunting first thing can give you a disproportionate sense of satisfaction and resolve for the rest of the day.

I prefer to call them 'bears', based on Michael Rosen's classic children's book *We're Going on a Bear Hunt*, with the inescapable refrain on each page recognising that we're just going to have to tackle every obstacle in our path and go through it: a mantra for daily life.

Richard Koch's seminal bestseller *The 80/20 Principle* dedicates his book to one simple premise: that 20 per cent of what we do accounts for 80 per cent of the impact. It's another powerful argument to rid ourselves of the incidental tasks and zone in on that one crucial thing – be it frog, rock or bear. 'Think about the biggest impact you can have in the smallest amount of time. Confine it to something that won't take longer than an hour and concentrate on doing that, then put your feet up,' says Koch.

Each week, sit down with a pen and paper and write down

two – to cover both productivity days – of the 'frogs', 'rocks' or 'bears' that you can't go over or under but must go through.

Now you need to combine these heavy tasks with a time in your day when you feel at your sharpest. 'I'm a great believer in managing our work by our attention and energy levels,' says Graham Allcott. A growing body of research suggests (see Productivity Facts, p.152) that paying attention to our body clock can help us focus on when we feel most productive. Most of us, according to Steve Kay, a professor of molecular and computational biology at the University of Southern California, are cognitively at our best in late morning. Body temperature starts to rise just before we wake up and increase through to midday, as do alertness and concentration. Taking a warm morning shower can boost these natural rhythms.

Certainly some of the world's greatest minds did apply themselves early each morning, from Mozart to Georgia O'Keeffe to Frank Lloyd Wright, according to a book about the productivity habits of famous achievers, *Daily Rituals* by Mason Currey. But everyone is different, so think about your typical working day and the peaks of your concentration: when they occur, how long they last. Now reflect on when would be the best or worst time to complete a demanding task.

Allcott defines different attention levels as:

- Proactive – those two or three golden hours when your concentration is at its peak.

- Active – when your concentration is less razor-sharp but not yet dulled.

- Inactive – the tail end of your concentration when you're almost running on empty but able to thrive on more automated tasks.

Now look at your 'rocks' list and think about combining that golden window of proactivity with those chunky, energy-demanding tasks.

> *My usual way of working is to leave everything to the last minute and then power through it at top speed. I feel lethargic when I'm putting things off and full of energy when I'm actually knuckling down to it. I then look back and think that if I worked at that level all the time I'd be a millionaire. So now I set myself personal deadlines – I may have a week to finish something but I give myself two days. When that's done I move on to the next thing and find I am getting a lot more done. My big obstacle is picking up the phone – I would much rather email, but then find myself stalled waiting for the reply. I now make myself call to keep things flowing. I worry about being a nuisance but tell myself that isn't the case, I'm a valuable member of the team.*
>
> Jo, 47

> *I have been putting off writing up the financial section of a work report but when I finally get down to breaking it down into manageable chunks it feels much more achievable. The worst part has been not knowing how much work it will entail, how great the demands will be. Once I draw up a plan, get it down on paper, talk it through with a colleague and make a timeframe, I feel much better.*
>
> Jenny, 30

David Allen refers to this relief as 'getting it out of your head.' 'Nothing changed in your world except how you engaged in the world. Your psyche is a little office full of strange machinations, which is why you need to get stuff out of there. Once you can do this, your mind is a much better place to exist.'

My morning ritual used to be: drop the kids off, get to work and, for the first hour, check my emails, look at Facebook and Twitter and generally surf the net. I know I've wasted valuable time basically skiving, but I've managed to persuade myself it's my way of gearing up to work. Trouble is, there's not much time left to actually do it! So now I write a list of five things I need to do that day and tell myself that if I do at least three of them I can reward myself with Facebook for fifteen minutes before carrying on. The joy of crossing each one out as I do it is so satisfying.

Louise, 30

Try 5:2 as a daily ratio

We know that the 5:2 approach works well as a weekly balance but it also echoes the rhythm of our working day too.

'You can choose your two productivity days but also break that down a step further,' suggests Allcott. 'As in changing or introducing a new habit for two out of a seven-hour working day.'

You don't need to focus on your heavyweight mental tasks in this two-hour window. It could include a number of self-discipline techniques (see Step 7) that can aid what you're already doing. Or try this:

For two hours out of every seven of your working day, don't check emails or go online. Allcott punctuates his working day with consciously being on- and offline to boost productivity. 'My regular pattern is to be on the internet between 8 and 9 a.m. to mainly check the news and current events. Then I'm off between 9 a.m and 1 p.m. when I'm tackling the decision-making and creative tasks. In the afternoon I'm 'on' internet and email until I finish work – that's my collaborative time when I'm doing meetings, emailing and making calls. So for half of Allcott's day, he 'goes dark'. 'Once you take emails out you have an amazing focus for other things,' he says.

For two hours each day, could you go dark? It may feel unrealistic at first but, for many of us, it really isn't. Think about those two-hour meetings or working lunches when screen time isn't a burning priority. Apart from getting more done, this simple constraint will make you more thoughtful about your online activity, keener to curb and control those urges and impulses.

'The first thing people do is turn on Outlook and it stays on all day. Ask them to turn it off and they freak,' says Allcott. It's like a security blanket that we can't imagine life without but, once you do, it makes you think in a slightly different way. 'I started to think ahead more when I knew I couldn't use email for a while, and felt more aware of when and why I was using it.'

I love receiving emails and it is a welcome break from work to check them but actually they are distracting me and breaking my concentration, so I tried not checking them for two hours each day. Instead of having my inbox visible in my menu bar on my computer, I hid it so didn't see when new ones arrived. I also turned my email notification to silent on my phone. It was scary to realise quite how often I reflexively look at the bottom left corner of my screen, expecting to see my Hotmail menu bar. At first I felt worried that I might miss something that needed an instant reply but discovered that if someone needed to know something urgently they followed it up with a phone call. I don't banter as much with colleagues via email but that's probably a good thing!

Ben, 29

6 Make your weekends sacred

We know that 5:2 is a versatile ratio that can be applied within the working day as well as across two productivity days each week. In this step, however, 5:2 takes on a different emphasis, referring to five working days and the importance of a two-day weekend break.

As our screen life becomes ever more compelling or intrusive, depending on how you feel about it, and as work time, social media and free time are merged ever further, the traditional concept of the weekend has shifted radically. All-day shopping, twenty-four-hour culture and communication, continually checking tweets, emails and texts across the weekend has blurred the traditional 5:2 divide.

'We're increasingly willing to sacrifice our weekends because we're living in challenged times and feel we have to work more to be "connected". Twitter and Facebook can make us feel productive when really there's very little being done,' says Allcott.

Be aware of boundaries – do you tend to let work bleed into weekends? Do you reflexively check work emails either on your phone or screen?

Here's how you can ring-fence your weekend:

1) Turn your work screen and laptops off – keep them in a separate room if necessary. Go into the settings on your mobile phone – and tablet if applicable – and turn off your work email account for Saturday and Sunday.

2) Be conscious of switching off from work at the end of each work day. Make a list at the end of each day to reassure yourself that it's okay to leave the office at a set time – don't delay it. This will help you be firmer about fencing in Saturday and Sunday too.

145

As Tony Schwarz, time-management expert (see Step 7 below) says, 'Prioritising itself turns out to require time. Part of my evening ritual is to take five to thirty minutes before I leave my office every day to sort through what I've done that day, and decide what makes most sense to begin with the next.'

3) Don't feel guilty about this complete break from everything work related. Instead feel guilty if you fail to take time out. Allcott says, 'No way will I touch a list between Friday and Monday morning. This isn't taking time off, it's about increasing productivity for the rest of the time. Any work that requires adding value to information requires analysis and focus. Only a rested brain can achieve that.'

Remind yourself that you owe it to your boss to be at your most productive which means, according to extensive research, working no more than forty hours each week with a complete two-day rest. Evidence? The law of diminishing returns. Henry Ford famously cut shifts at his car production plants from nine to eight hours because, after years of study, he found the formula for optimum productivity was 5:2. They discovered that forty hours each week is the ideal – when they added another twenty hours there was a minor increase in productivity, but only for three to four weeks before productivity levels declined.

4) Make a to-do list on Friday evening of where you want to start on Monday morning so you know exactly where to jump in and you feel more relaxed walking away from your desk before the weekend.

I work between my office and home, and I know the dangers of letting business seep into weekend time. I close my laptop down early Friday evening and it goes into my work bag and stays in the corner of my room until Monday morning. I work for an international company and clients do email over the weekend. Yes, I am tempted to check up on stuff but then I tell myself it's my responsibility to manage my time well, give myself distance and come back refreshed to give them, and my managers, the best I can.

Daniel, 34

Since doing 5:2 Your Screen Life, I make sure that the weekend is a time to stay away from screens and devices which means cultural activities on my own or with my kids, usually that I've searched out and planned ahead – trips to museums, art galleries, special screenings and theatre matinees – something to look forward to that is an alternative experience to take us away from the default setting of languishing on sofas staring at screens or checking my email!

Harry, 49

⑦ 'Tabata' your workload

If you've read 5:2 Your Fitness, you'll know that Professor Izumi Tabata helped to pioneer high-intensity interval workouts (HIIT), along with other sports scientists since. Using this technique during exercise, people push themselves to the extreme for a minute or two, take time out to recover, then repeat – with significant health benefits.

Experts believe that pushing ourselves physically in brief but intense bursts, much like denying the body food in the 5:2 diet, is an extremely efficient way of boosting the body's productivity. As I described earlier in this chapter, transferring this technique to work feels like a no-brainer – as Tony Schwarz, CEO of the

Energy Project and time management expert, worked out long before I did, thanks to his running routine. He began running at higher speeds in short intervals of thirty and sixty seconds, resting for the same amount of time between: his interval workout is only seven to ten minutes in total. Schwarz now applies the interval approach to his work and business. 'I start by doing the most important thing first for ninety minutes, then I take a break between fifteen to thirty minutes. That's the right amount of time (see research in Productivity Facts, p.152).'

Renewal is key, he says. The more he switches off, the more relaxed he feels afterwards. At his offices, employees can unwind in a 'renewal room'. They also finish work at 6 p.m. and switch off email over evenings and weekends – respecting the 5:2 weekend rule.

On one of your two productivity days each week, Tabata your workload, ideally applying this intensive burst to the most important task of the day for ninety minutes at a time. Key to your success is recognising that if you don't find it taxing and challenging, you're not working hard enough – just like the seven-minute workout. At the same time, these feelings of discomfort will pass quickly and you can look forward to relaxation and recovery afterwards. Walking around the office, or outside if possible, for even five minutes is physically beneficial and gives you a screen break – it also counts as worthwhile incidental exercise as outlined in 5:2 Your Fitness.

Running at high-intensity intervals can be exhausting, discovered Schwarz, and it's the same with work productivity. But the payoffs are immense, as he says, 'I've built these principles into the way I write. For my first three books, I sat at my desk for up to ten hours a day. Each of the books took me at least a year to write. For my two most recent books, I wrote in three uninterrupted ninety-minute sessions each day – beginning first thing in the morning, when my energy was highest – and took a break after each one.'

You might want to build up to the Tabata method and try the Pomodoro technique first, invented by Francesco Cirillo. You'll need a kitchen timer – Cirillo uses one shaped like a tomato, which gives this exercise its name. Set the timer for twenty-five minutes and try to apply yourself to the task in hand with the same intense vigour as you would to running a race; all-out effort to see how far you can get by the time your timer rings. No diversion, no distraction, think only of that timer and what you can achieve in less than half an hour. Rest for five minutes after each twenty-five-minute interlude. Repeat three more times and allow yourself a longer break.

I Pomodoro my son and daughter's morning routine now – I think Tabata may be a bit extreme for them! Getting ready for school is usually so stressful because they need constant nagging to get out of bed. So now it's a timed challenge with reward points that convert into treats out. I give them twenty-five minutes to get dressed, downstairs and eat their breakfast. It really motivates them and makes it into a fun game. My 11-year-old son also does his homework in twenty-five-minute chunks too, with small rests between – it's a good amount of time for a child to really focus and concentrate and he likes the novelty of the red tomato ticking away.
Tom, 48

I tried both the twenty-five-minute and ninety-minute techniques and although I thought I'd prefer the shorter one, I discovered that it was actually too short for the type of work

I do. I design websites and to really get stuck in, I need a good hour and a half. But overall, knowing that I am going full steam ahead for a limited time encourages me to be effective.'
Matthew, 38

You may wonder why not just get on and do it anyway? Schwarz says, 'When something is open-ended, with no defined period of time, and that goes for exercise too, you won't be fully engaged.' Therein lies the central attraction for me – anything is possible when it ends soon.

When you can see and feel the physical benefits of HIIT, and a 5:2 fast day if you've tried it, you'll know those same benefits will quickly come about if you 5:2 Your Productivity too.

Going for a very fast, but very brief run in the mornings is far more manageable than trying to find an hour twice a week – even if I come back looking like a pomodoro. So trying it with work too was a revelation. With my usual workload, I'd space things out over the day – this after lunch, this at 4 p.m., and so on. Instead I crammed as much as I could in the first half-hour and was amazed. I felt like the bionic woman and that I really deserved my morning coffee break.
Ruth, 32

COMMON QUESTIONS

Which two days should I choose to focus on 5:2 productivity?

Cut the 5:2 ratio two ways and apply to two nonconsecutive weekdays. Also bear in mind the 5:2 approach every weekend to remind yourself that these two days should be a sanctuary from – not an overflow for – your working week.

What should I bear in mind for the other five days?

Using two working days to focus on bursts of intense productivity will inevitably influence your other days too. Expect to achieve more by Friday afternoon and feel calmer and more rested by Monday morning.

Which other 5:2 life areas combine well with productivity?

  5:2 Your **Fitness** is an ideal companion. Putting high-intensity exercise and high-intensity work back-to-back is even better, as I discovered. Experiment in other areas of your life – Tabata your vacuuming, your walk or cycle ride to work, but definitely not your driving!

5:2 Your **Productivity** is a natural fit with 5:2 Your **Screen Life** – annexing weekends to make them email free, as well as turning emails off for two hours on your working days, makes you more mindful when you log back in.

You can also try the mindful meditation exercises (on p.219 of 5:2 Your **Worry**) during your Tabata rest periods. Making lists and decluttering your inbox will also help to reduce overall work stress.

PRODUCTIVITY FACTS

- In 2011, a study at the University of Illinois followed two groups of participants completing a repetitive computerised task. One worked without diversion for fifty minutes, the other 'switch' group was allowed to take two brief breaks to concentrate on something else. The first group's concentration declined significantly during the hour while the 'switch' group saw no drop in performance. 'We propose that deactivating and reactivating your goals allows you to stay focused,' said psychology professor Alejandro Lleras, who led the study.

- An hour and a half is the most effective length of time to work for, according to Florida State University. In a study of elite performers including actors, musicians and sportspeople, they discovered that the best performers were those who limited themselves to ninety-minute uninterrupted intervals and only four-and-a-half hours a day. Dr Phil Race, an expert on effective learning, says that those short periods of enforced inactivity, such as your daily commute, are a great opportunity to teach yourself something as your brain is receptive to stimulus, and small bursts of learning sink in better.

- A paper by the European Foundation for the Improvement of Living and Working Conditions reveals that among the sixteen of the EU nations, people who worked more flexible hours or jobs that would be normally considered part-time were overall more engaged with and productive at work and happier in their leisure time than people who worked more hours.

- It's easy to assume that morning is the best time to tackle the heavy stuff, but according to a 2011 study published in the journal *Thinking & Reasoning*, there is no hard-and-fast rule – the key is to work the hours that are best for you.

5:2

YOUR SCREEN LIFE

LIFE BEFORE MY 5:2 SCREEN LIFE DIET

This time last year technology was taking over my household. At first it was amusing, the sight of my three children bunched up on the sofa, aged 11, 9 and 2, arms and legs entwined, in tablet heaven: the eldest on his iPad mini, the middle on her iPod Touch, and the youngest on my iPad.

On any weekend morning, everywhere I looked there would be evidence of heavy usage, with earphone wires and socket extensions trailing across the floor. 'I need my next charge,' my 11-year-old son would insist, whenever his iPad threatened to flatline and the battery level slip below 10 per cent. Meanwhile my 2-year-old would slump in dejection when her favourite TV programme on the iPad faded away, a signal for me to scrabble around for a lead before there was an iTantrum.

This, then, was my increasingly seven-day-a-week iFamily; one where our leisure time was to a great extent shaped by tablets, phones and laptops – either by Apple or its proliferating rivals – and where much of our communication was characterised by the following:

Eldest: What's your password for iTunes again?

Middle: Mum, she's just deleted the LOVEFiLM app!

Youngest: iPad gone black. [Cries.]

So it went on.

It all felt like new territory for me. When my two elder children were born, I had a television, mobile phone and a highly child-unfriendly computer. They would watch certain DVDs over and over again, but that was it.

Ten years later, my youngest responded so instinctively to a touch-screen, she would stroke every flat surface expectantly, and still does, waiting for it to light up and activate. 'Look, iPad waking up again,' she'd say whenever the Apple logo pulsed seductively back to life.

Digital dependency

Another Saturday morning and the children are huddled on the sofa plugged into their screens, accompanied to a clashing chorus of soundtracks dredged from all corners of the internet. I slope into the kitchen where my husband and I retreat and tune out into a similarly addictive digital world of online news, emails and social media. This is our downtime, a leisurely way into the weekend, so why do I feel dissatisfied?

I know that part of this problem is about shared dependency; as much as I criticise my children's usage, it suits me too – I can only really blame myself. I've just bought a new laptop and smartphone and I'm enthralled with – and hooked on – both. My addiction is their addiction, so what right do I have to complain?

As a parent, I feel guilty because I know I should be monitoring and imposing many more rules than I do. Instead I resort to exasperated threats, shrieking at them when it's time for homework, bath or guitar practice. With the communal joys of FaceTime, Apple's version of Skype, my lame rants and outbursts are often witnessed in real time with great amusement by a bunch of their friends, and parents too for all I know.

I'm extremely aware that family conflict in our household tends to erupt when I've allowed the children to languish for too long on screens. I vent my guilt and frustration, usually with impotent threats to throw away their chargers, a negative cycle that plays out too often.

Partly I resist being too stringent because, clearly, I enjoy the window of freedom this shared technology affords. Having a toddler third time round isn't the same deal at all – long car journeys are less fraught. Reading a newspaper feature uninterrupted is no longer in the realm of fantasy, but I wonder at what price.

Something had to change

Our family's digital habits were not unusual or even extreme, that much was clear. Around this time, there were scare stories of children unwittingly racking up thousands of pounds' worth of debt on their parents' accounts, making app-purchases without authorisation. One four-year-old girl was in the news when her parents admitted her to a clinic for compulsive behaviour therapy; she had become increasingly 'distressed and inconsolable' when her screen was taken away, using it up to four hours a day.

These weren't typical examples but, even so, I would compare notes with other mothers and wonder, should we ban them altogether, and if so, just for weekends or for weeks at a time? And should we lead by example and unplug our phones and laptops too?

I began to pine for the monolithic charms of the television – only one remote to control, one voice, TV programme or soundtrack. Bliss, I reflected, compared to this scenario, where as soon as I turned my back, another screen popped up, yet another window and volume button with a squawking, tinny soundtrack.

When our 10-year-old begged us for a tablet the Christmas before last, we caved in, partly because we were seduced too. Parents are as childishly enthralled as their teenage sons and tiny babies, which is why these devices have infiltrated home life on such an unprecedented scale – over 100 million iPads alone, let alone tablet PCs, were sold worldwide by 2012.

Even now, as a Screen Life Diet evangelist, I can still see my daughter's joy at controlling what she consumes with a fingertip, right there and then. While she happily navigates her way around the iPlayer and sends out the odd accidental tweet via her favourite Japanese game app, her grandma sits next to her on her own iPad watching repeats of *Pointless*.

But by last year, the novelty began to wane. The lack of interaction when most members of our household were online was spooky; there was no conversation, arguing or laughter. I wasn't exactly a great role model, checking my emails and Twitter feed while they did their homework. I wanted to alter our habits but I wasn't exactly sure when or how. I didn't want our family routine to transform radically, but we needed more boundaries and rules, more discussion on how to control this new technology rather than being passively in thrall to it.

I'd read about Digital Detox, popular in the US: remote retreats where you have leave all your devices at home, with the slogan 'Disconnect to reconnect'.

But what happens when you do 'reconnect'? I couldn't see how this sort of approach would fit into the context of real life back at home. Besides, total abstinence isn't part of my nature, nor my children's for that matter. I know that technology is integral to modern family life, whatever we may feel about it, and that banning it wouldn't benefit my children in the long run. Much better, I felt, to embrace screens and devices, however intrusive they may seem, and aim for moderation. Exercising restraint in an achievable way was an ideal, and I continued to ponder quite how to attain it when, along with so many others, I decided to try the 5:2 diet.

MAKING THE 5:2 CONNECTION

That's when I made the link. A few weeks into the diet, and already impressed by its results, I began to wonder if a similar approach would work well for our screen lives too. Its moderate premise means it's well suited to a child's natural temperament. How much more palatable from their point of view, to hear, 'No, you can't do this today but you can have as much as you want, within reason, tomorrow.'

Why not, then, a sensible technology fast where they could cut down rather than go cold turkey? Actually, 5:2 isn't that lukewarm – it works out as almost 20 per cent less food each week. In screen terms, that's an awful lot less CBeebies and Minecraft.

I approached Dr Richard Graham, child and adolescent psychiatrist at London's Tavistock Clinic and Capio Nightingale Hospital, who launched the first technology-addiction programme three years ago, and here offers his advice in my seven steps to make the screen diet work for you. He was extremely encouraging when I told him about the 5:2 blueprint and could see immediately how helpful it could be for our screen habits too.

The 5:2 approach isn't extreme and yet it still allows sufficient space to give yourself pause for reflection. As Professor Rose Luckin, professor of learner-centred design at the University of London, says, 'For so many of us, including families, this could be a great way of achieving a balance. It's restrictive when it needs to be but also offers you freedom. When you go back to your screen life, you'll appreciate and savour what you watch a lot more.'

THE 5:2 SCREEN LIFE DIET; aims and benefits

- The Screen Life Diet takes the tools of the 5:2 food diet, improving habits twice a week to benefit the other five.

- It helps you to cut down the amount of television you watch, as well as time spent on PCs, laptops, PlayStation and mobiles.

- The principle is easy to communicate to children of all ages – taking away screens for two days a week is a simple, black-and-white rule. This is not a digital detox or a total ban; they – and you – are never more than twenty-four hours away from your favourite programme or app.

- A two-day screen fast offers a great window to initiate new family activities, especially if you choose one weekend day. The time away will demand that you reflect more about what technology you use and why.

- You and your children will be happier; this is a shared project where you will enjoy more time with each other, be more mindful, in the moment, and engaged as a family.

GETTING STARTED ON THE 5:2 SCREEN LIFE DIET

Abstinence is not the answer, especially where children are involved. They will engage with technology whatever rules you impose now. But, while they're young, you have a window of opportunity, with the help of the 5:2 philosophy, to build in sensible rules and attitudes.

Now you've read my experience and why I decided to apply 5:2 dieting to my family's screen life, you'll want to know how to make it work for you. These seven steps will outline how to plan for a Screen Life Diet, what to expect, and how your screen-fast habits can fit flexibly into daily family life.

SEVEN STEPS TO MAKE THE 5:2 SCREEN LIFE DIET WORK FOR YOU

1

Do a screen audit
Studies suggest that dieters who make a record tend to be more successful – once you get it down on paper, it somehow feels more concrete. When I first started the 5:2 diet, I bought two sets of scales, one for the kitchen and one for the bathroom. So it is with the Screen Life Diet, you need to measure your usage to know how much you want to reduce it by.

Sit down with your family, draw a column for each member of the family and take notes.

'Talking about it is critical to the outcome I think', says Dr Richard Graham. 'Learning to be mindful about your relationship with technology will always effect change. When I'm talking about this in schools I'll often start a discussion with "Where did you first go online?" and we build a timeline of use – it's a real icebreaker in the process of thinking about how we use screens.'

Professor Luckin agrees. 'In all the time I've been studying technology and family, the most overwhelmingly successful approach is when you open it up with your children, find out how it works, understand what's good and bad and all engage with it.'

Technology and screen time isn't exclusively a family issue. If you don't have children, use this time to talk about your personal tastes, habits and preferences with your partner or friend, or you can reflect on your own and record what you use, when and why; essential as a cornerstone to the other steps.

This can't be an exact science, like standing on the scales, but try and map out a realistic picture. Here are some questions you could include:

- How many hours a day do each of us spend on our screens? List everything from television and DVDs to PlayStations and Nintendo DS, tablets, PCs, laptops and mobile phones.

- What's your favourite activity online, and why?

- What about social media – which type do you use most?

- Can you give a rough breakdown of your activities, e.g. 50 per cent checking emails and texts, 50 per cent online window shopping?

- When are the 'hotspot' times for usage – after work or school, morning or after tea?

- When are you most drawn to go online? When you're bored? Tired? Feeling antisocial? Draw out any emotional triggers, if possible, for parents and children.

Which one are you?

In June 2013, researchers at Northwestern University in the US released a survey that divides families into three types: 'media-light' families, where parents use screens for less than two hours a day and children less than 1.5 hours; 'media-moderate' families, where the usage is just under five and three hours a day respectively; and 'media-centric' families, where the usage in each case is 11 hours and 4.5 hours.

'There is a trickiness in trying to capture your usage accurately', says Dr Graham. 'How do you measure it if you text while watching TV while checking your emails? But that doesn't matter, because whatever you come up with tells us something, builds a picture and gets you thinking.'

For Step 1 of the process, our screen audit, I sit with a pad and go through each family member in turn. We agree that parents' screen use during work hours is exempt, but we still have to be honest about time spent internet surfing; window shopping online, etc. Similarly, online research for children's homework is fine, too, but needs to be monitored.

Initially the children are slightly defensive, as if they've been called to the headmaster's office. Eldest: 'Er, I don't want to say how long I spend in case it makes me look bad.' Middle: 'Definitely less than an hour a day. Is that the end of the discussion?' After further coaxing, we conclude 1.5 hours each on a weekday for all three children, rising to 2.5 hours at weekends, more including a family film in the evening. My evening usage can be categorised as: DVD box sets and obsessively checking work email and texts, plus a worrying amount of online window shopping, weighing in at around two hours a day too; it's a similar picture for my husband.

I ask them more generally what they like about going online and reassure them we're not going to be judgemental or tell them off. Within ten minutes they warm to explaining what they like and why. I'm aware that although this is a significant activity in their lives, we never share it in a positive way, it tends to get dismissed by their parents and criticised as a pointless activity.

'They have a hunger to open up about it, maybe because of the gap between our generation and theirs', says Dr Graham. 'For so many parents, what their children enjoy online just doesn't resonate – it's hard to understand their world, which is why this is such a useful exercise. It also paves the way to raise other serious issues later, about nasty images online or cyber-bullying.'

The principles of the 5:2 approach to diet mean that you're slashing calorie intake by around 20 per cent per week. However, on our screen diet days, the idea is that usage falls to almost zero except for Saturday evening television. That's around 33 per cent less time online over the week as a whole, a much healthier balance.

At first I was apprehensive about doing this with our family and charting an average week; a bit like the dread of getting on the scales and facing your worst fears. It was a really interesting exercise, though, sharing what the kids like about

going online for the first time. And we could immediately see the blackspots – early evening before tea when the two girls go onto Facebook and I'll endlessly check my emails and texts.
    Katherine, 42

This turned into such an interesting discussion – my children are 10 and 12 years old and, as a working parent, I'm quick to dismiss what they watch as low-quality rubbish, but when they talked about the different programmes and websites they enjoyed, I began to see it very differently. They're picky and discerning about what they consume, they're thoughtful about the stuff they see – that felt like a worthwhile thing to discover.
    Kate, 38

2 Set the rules

Be firm about what is on and off limits on your Screen Life Diet days – include this as part of your screen audit. The more you clarify now, the less you'll need to troubleshoot later on. Make it watertight.

Each individual and family is different and so what you decide to exclude on your Screen Life Diet day will vary. This is fine – 5:2 is about aiming for what you feel is realistic and achievable, not overstretching.

You may want to start by cutting down to only thirty minutes online two days a week and then increasing that time over a month. It's up to you as long as it gives you enough space to create new offline activities and feel the difference.

You may decide that FaceTime is fine but texting isn't, or vice versa, depending on your habits. What's more important is sticking to the perimeters, whatever they are, once you've agreed them.

Early on we faced two dilemmas; as a working parent at home, I still needed to check some emails and texts every day and the children had to do some of their homework online. I also want to combine my 5:2 Fitness Plan with Screen Life Diet days – the only problem is that means using my iPhone as it's got my playlists and a podcast, which both motivate me to run.

Dr Graham had some advice. 'Firstly I'd say, I think you need to make a judgement call between constructive and nonconstructive emails and texts; the ones that relate to initiating offline activities, which I think are fine, and conversational ones that are more social – those should be ignored. And only very important work emails,' he suggests. 'In terms of homework, I would say on screen-fast days this is also fine to do online but needs to be monitored by a parent – ideally at the kitchen table.' Consequently, I agreed with the family that I was allowed to take my iPhone running, but no sneakily sending texts after I ran around the block.

Here's what our house rules looked like:

- On Thursdays, zero screen activity. For children, this means no laptops or PCs, no iPod Touches or TV. No email, texting or FaceTime.

- All mobile devices to be stored away together to reduce chances of temptation – out of sight, out of mind.

- Adults, outside office hours, no PC, laptop or tablets. Check phones sparingly, ideally away from children, for important calls and texts.

- On Saturdays, buy newspapers rather than read online.

- Zero screen activity until evening – family television or film.

We got a blackboard in our kitchen and it helped to map out what would be happening every Tuesday and Thursday – we'd write a list of what was strictly off limits and asked them to list any activities they'd like to do. We made sure they realised this wasn't only a two-week experiment – but a subtle and permanent change to our life.

Sally, 34

When I introduced the two-day screen diet to my 11-year-old daughter, I spoke to the mothers of some of her friends who often text, email and FaceTime each other in the evenings – we agreed to coincide the same two days off and try it together so none of them felt they were missing out.

Janice, 45

Usually my iPhone is with me all the time, I feel as if I've lost a limb if it isn't; my boyfriend feels the same way about his laptop. But for two evenings a week we leave them upstairs. One aspect I really don't miss is the continual soundtrack of beeps, vibrations and ringtones that take over our home these days. I'm really appreciative of that silence.

Daisy, 28

3 Set goals

Think about where you'd all like to be in four weeks' time and write down one goal. If applicable, ask your children to suggest one positive experience they hope to gain from the two-day screen diet – it could be something as simple as 'More cycle rides with Dad.' Or create your own list of potential benefits. Keep these somewhere safe and check them after one month on your screen diet to measure your progress.

'It's a good way to make them feel they'll be gaining a genuine reward for giving something up, an experience that they can savour that's a bit more memorable than watching something online,' says Graham.

Here are what my family's goals looked like:

- Me: 'In one month's time, I want our two-day Screen Life Diet to be so much a part of our family rhythm we don't even notice it. I know this isn't a major change but I want it to feel substantial enough that I won't want to return to our pre-diet screen life.'

- Husband: 'This will only be worth it if it improves our screen days too, so that I'll finally be able to use my own iPad without having to fight off a small child.'

- Eldest: 'I'd like Dad to finally get that backgammon board down from the loft.'

- Middle: 'I love reading, and being read to, and I want to finish *Little Women* with Mum in the evenings. We always run out of time.'

Also start thinking of more positive ways you can engage with technology for the rest of the week. 'Think about how to make use of these devices in a creative way: cameras, videos, editing apps, online board games, all sorts of possibilities to explore together,' says Professor Luckin. Aim to avoid the 'us and them' isolated scenario of children and parents or partners online in separate rooms. 'Who else is involved when you're online? Are most members of your family solitary users? How can you change this?'

I'm so much more aware now of how my 20-month-old toddler uses the iPad; how it can be constructive when I'm there but so much less so when I leave her to it; there's such a difference letting her watch Dumbo *alone compared to sitting next to her, chatting about it, pointing stuff out and enjoying it together.*

Louisa, 40

I live on my own and find myself ever more dependent on social media – texting and answering emails at midnight. It's as if I can't switch off, trying to think of the next witty tweet to write when I should be reading and falling asleep. It's a constant urge to be distracting myself, in "doing" mode. I tell myself it's a good way of relaxing and yet it takes a surprising amount of brain power, it's not a brilliant way of winding down, really. And I don't even get that lovely engaged feeling you enjoy with a good film or book. It's just a habit though. I wonder what I'm really avoiding sometimes. I'd like to test myself and find out.

Jenny, 30

If you're thinking of goals, a trip to the local library and reading as a family is perhaps the best one of all. According to a National Literacy Trust study in September 2012, of 21,000 children and teenagers, only three in every ten read daily in their own time, down from four in ten in 2005.

On weekend mornings, there's no screen time and my husband and I sit and read to our two boys, 6 and 8 years old; the one activity that falls off our to-do list because screens get in the way.

Trish, 38

4. Think about quality, not just quantity

Your attitude to technology should mirror your relationship to food. You need a balanced diet of interaction on- and offline. Those YouTube clips and apps that you and your family enjoy are fine, just like the odd plate of chips. But think about more balance and 'nutrition'; more National Geographic and BBC for every viral video. 'It's a good comparison to draw,' says Luckin. 'Some games and programmes are more like fast food rather than a nice meal – pay attention to keeping their screen diet richer and more 'nutritious' on the other five days.'

If you have children, ask them to explain their choices and take time to be curious about what they watch and enjoy, so you can make more informed choices about their consumption, as well as your own.

I always worried how consumed my two elder children were by the hugely popular building game Minecraft. Unchallenged, they would play it twelve hours each day. During the times they were using it, I would often berate them for being unresponsive and unaware, while I grew crosser by the minute. In our screen-free space, I've got their full attention and we talk more about why they enjoy Minecraft. I'm less judgemental and they're more articulate about why they like it. One reason is they're able to share and play on it together; they want me to go on too so they can show me how to play, prove to me how creative it can be.

For the first time I notice how these two days away from screens are defining and shaping our days online. I factor in time now to talk about how we use our screens, how the children feel when they see me constantly monitoring texts and emails, and how we could share online activities more.

At first quantity was the real issue for us, which is why we tried this out in the first place, but as we got into it more, and talked to the children about what they like online, we became far more aware of quality, of negotiating with them on their onscreen days much more about what they watch, rather than just how much.

Richard, 50

5 Make a plan

The day before your first day without screens or technology, plan your activities and get the whole family involved. If it's a school or work day, homework and limited hours in the evening will help fill that time for you, but on a long Saturday or Sunday a plan is helpful, especially in the first week or two.

'Try to plan activities outside the home as much as possible,' suggests Graham. 'To give yourself less distraction from chores and thoughts of going online too.'

If applicable, ask your children to suggest one thing they'd really like to do – if they can't agree, plot out on the calendar how each day might look. The more involved children are in the timetable, the more willing they will be to stick to it. Or you might create a list just to please yourself!

This is what our activity plan looked like;

Thursdays
  Park after school. Reading/homework. Tea. Table tennis match. Reading. Bed.

Saturday
  Morning: Different family activities including swimming, and cycling in the park. Reading for one hour – non-negotiable. Lunch.

Afternoon: free exhibition at museum/art gallery.
Evening: cook meal with help of children. Film/family television.

6 Change the scene

Staring at a flat surface for long periods of time doesn't challenge all our senses, or give the brain all that it needs. This is even more reason to get physical on your screen-fast days – away from temptation but also exerting your mind and body in a different and contrasting way.

Physical

Factor in at least one physical activity on your Screen Life Diet days – something as simple as a fifteen-minute walk around your local park. Swimming, cycling and running are ideal too.

'This isn't about activity as distraction,' says Dr Graham. 'It's drawing on your body in a different way, using your physical self on those days off and noticing how different it feels – focus on other senses too.'

Mental

Like healthy snacks in the fridge to deter you from high-calorie grazing, keep board games like solitaire and backgammon set up, ready to play, or gather together books or articles you've been meaning to read.

Give your children a drawing challenge – a week to complete an assignment like, 'Your Home Town in the 25th Century' and offer a good incentive to win, like a trip to the cinema or favourite pizzeria.

Encourage them to practice a musical instrument even twice a week – many studies studies link music study to academic achievement. In a recent article in the *New York Times*, writer

Joanne Lipman talked to professionals who were also dedicated musicians. All of them linked their success to their musical experience in some way, suggesting a relationship between music and other key attributes – the ability to work as part of a team, to listen and focus in different ways, to think more laterally and creatively: benefits a screen can more rarely offer you.

> *We finally caved in to pressure and bought ourselves a trampoline for our two sons. Now it's so easy distracting them during those offscreen hours, it almost feels like cheating!*
> Joanna, 44

Our first family screen diet day coincides with half-term. Twelve hours yawn ahead of us. I have turned off my phone and computer, stashed away all the children's devices, unplugged the TV and hidden the remotes. We are officially a family offline. The house is weirdly silent. There's only one way out. I book three tickets to the cinema. It means leaving home and doing something we all enjoy, but it is also one huge screen. I call Dr Graham to check I'm not cheating. 'Fine,' he says. 'It's a different sensory experience and it's something you're sharing together. On the downside, the film you've chosen has rather mixed reviews.'

I leave my youngest at home with a childminder under strict instructions keep all devices hidden and stick to *Where's Spot?* 'To make this watertight, there must be no weak links,' Dr Graham advises. No indulgent grandmas, partners or nannies. And no cheating if you're doing this on your own.

7   Be more mindful

Yes, the early days of screen fasting can be tough; dealing with tantrums from your toddler while fielding articulate objections from the older children isn't easy. It helps if you, and particularly children, can recognise that these feelings of frustration and restlessness are temporary.

At first my eldest feels the absence of screens the most. He is morose, restless, roaming from room to room like a caged lion. One daughter finger-paints, the other sculpts Fimo, but he can't let go. He forages through the kitchen drawer looking for a discarded mobile. I find him under a duvet upstairs on an old Nintendo game. I drag him downstairs to play chess. He reads, then chases his sister around the kitchen. It is tougher than I thought; we go to the park, play in the adventure playground, paddle in the pool – eking out those hours away from home, like alcoholics avoiding the pub – but it does help to talk about how we felt later that evening, understand that it's all transient

'From other areas of the addiction world, we know that the technique of noticing certain thoughts but not engaging with them can be very effective,' says Dr Graham. 'Reflect on those moments of agitation or craving but reassure yourself that they will pass and you'll feel better soon; the hopefulness of that belief will give you the strength to manage it.' You may find it helpful to refer to 5:2 Your Worry – the mindfulness meditations are an excellent way of observing moods and thoughts but not getting caught up by them (see p.219).

Professor Mark Williams advises, 'Whenever you or your family get that impulse to go online, to play games, check emails and texts, etc., rather than acting on it immediately, give yourself a fifteen-minute space. While you're doing it, notice how you feel; how does your body and mind respond?'

With some mindful reflection, I realise that experience is also key here to help sustain you; by the second week, the children know what to expect and it's less daunting. They find the rules easy to follow, as do I, and know that with famine today comes feast tomorrow.

My two eldest fight and argue; there's more noise and conflict, but we engage and discuss more too. They appreciate that I'm more involved with them, not continually checking my own emails and texts. They also both help me put their sister to bed and read to her when they'd normally be FaceTiming friends – a delightful benefit I hadn't predicted.

COMMON QUESTIONS

Why do I need to do this?

If you feel you rely too much on screen and technology, or that you're overwhelmed by the demands technology makes on your time, invading your space – the overflowing emails with Twitter alerts from people you don't know, prompts to update your Facebook account or connect with a stranger on LinkedIn. Or if you feel your children have become too dependent and, as a family, you enjoy fewer shared activities, all zoning out on different screens, this might be for you.

Which two days should I choose for my Screen Life Diet?

Ideally pick nonconsecutive days. As with the 5:2 diet, spreading the days out feels like less of an ordeal, crucial if you want to stick to the plan or have your children on board. Maybe start off gently at first, perhaps picking two weekdays if that feels like less of a jump, then move one day to a weekend.

Aim for rhythm that you feel you can get used to over time, that quickly feels like part of your routine.

I initially chose Mondays and Thursdays but, within a fortnight, I swapped my Monday to a Saturday to be able to plan more activities and appreciate more time feeling 'disconnected'.

Before you pick your days, tell people about it: friends, relations, mothers at the schools gates. If applicable, encourage your children to tell their friends too, so they'll understand why they can't respond to emails and texts for two days each week – once they, and you, go public, you'll cement that commitment.

What should I bear in mind for the other five days?

Just as the 5:2 diet encourages us to view food as a friend, not a foe, so it is with screens – this ratio allows us to enjoy what we consume but not in a habitual way; it would be self-defeating to fear and reject what gives us pleasure, and that includes technology too.

Establish in your or your child's mind that there are rules and limits seven days a week, not just on screen-fast days. These will vary depending on your child's age, but the first thing to emphasise is the framework.

However, ordering a child to turn off their computer can feel punitive, so whenever you encourage them to use it less, even on a screen day, try to encourage something positive they can do instead. Try suggesting an hour on the computer followed by switching it off for an hour, to give a sense of regulating their time online firmly but gently.

Which other 5:2 areas combine well with my Screen Life Diet?

Just as a drink and food fast are easy companions, matching your screen fast with your 5:2 **Fitness** Plan is logical too. Getting physical is a complete contrast to sitting staring at a PC, e-reader or device, challenging your body and brain in another way. As Professor Karen Pine, psychologist and author who advocates Doing Something Different (DSD) as a behavioural change technique, says, 'DSD works best when it's the opposite of your usual habit, to shake things up and challenge the status quo. In this way it can create a ripple effect across the week.'

Once I started, I discovered that combining my family screen diet with 5:2 Your Fitness worked really well for me. Early evening, when I would definitely have been online, I used that time to practice my ten-minute HIIT workout – because my 12-year-old son wasn't distracted by his screen, it's something we can do together now too.

*I also found my offline Saturdays meshed perfectly with 5:2 Your **Productivity** – keeping my weekends work-free and not checking emails. It made me reflect more when I was back on email – basically, how distracting they are when you want to get other things done. So I now have a two-hour email-free zone in my working day too, which I picked up from 5:2 Your Productivity.*

Dan, 33.

You might also consider doing your **Screen** Diet alongside the money-saving steps in 5:2 Your **Finance**: less time on-line means less opportunity to spend money or being lured by discount alerts. Your Screen Diet will also give you more time to spend with your partner as part of the 5:2 Your **Relationship** chapter – or at least more time together when you're not both on your phones!

What changes can I expect after a few weeks on a 5:2 Screen Life Diet?

Your household may well be noisier and more argumentative, but also less passive and self-absorbed, as mine now is. Like me, you may also feel as if you have a different family. For us, Thursdays and Saturdays are sacred: no FaceTime, texting, gaming, emailing or Twitter. I have bought a junior-size ping-pong table for the kitchen and there's a range of board games kept on the kitchen counter for easy access – backgammon, chess and solitaire; not unlike those 'healthy' treats I keep on standby on my fast days.

Best of all, my eldest is on board more each week. I ask him to compare fast days with feast ones. 'It's the difference between sitting on the sofa with a screen and you shouting at us all, or sitting at the kitchen table, drinking tea and chatting to you.'

I've discovered, as Luckin advises, screens and devices work best when we share activities: digesting and reading information for school projects, drawing and creating stuff together with art and animation apps. More generally, once you give yourself screen free days, or even chunks away from them each day, you'll become more aware of your online relationship. When you start to consciously check your emails and texts less often, take longer to reply, you'll discover they have less of a hold over you. You'll feel freer. And you'll begin to enjoy those spaces in between, feel less overwhelmed by the onslaught of emails and more in control of technology when you do decide to use it.

Hopefully, like me, you'll have discovered that a two-day screen void feels like a permanent life change and easy to maintain. It's not an extreme regime, more of a quiet revolution, which subtly transformed me and my family by kick-starting good habits and letting them spread.

At first I didn't like the idea at all when Mum and Dad first suggested it to us – I definitely didn't want to try it. I still find it tough, especially when I come home from school on Mondays, one of our days off, but it's nice to be able to share activities with Mum, rather than get told off for being on my iPad. I like that I only have to wait till tomorrow to play my favourite game, and that we talk more as a family.

Alex, 9

SCREEN LIFE FACTS

- According to Dr Aric Sigman, writing in the *Archives of Disease in Childhood*, the average 10-year-old has access to five different screens at home. A child born today will have spent the equivalent of a full year on screens by the time they reach the age of seven.

- In 2012, researchers at the University of Gothenburg studied the habits of more than 4,100 Swedish men and women aged between 20 and 24, and found that those who constantly use a computer or their mobile phone were more likely to develop sleeping disorders and depression. Lead author Sara Thomee said there was a 'central link' between computers and mental disorders. 'High quantitative use was a central link between computer use and stress, sleep disturbances, and depression,' she said.

- A quarter of British households now own at least one tablet, according to Ofcom, the communications regulator, and 91 per cent of those either allow their children to play with the device or have bought them one of their own. Games were the most used function at 71 per cent, followed by watching video clips and TV programmes. Two thirds of parents said tablets were useful when travelling.

- Although there has been widespread concern about the effects of text speak and abbreviation on a children's mastery of English language, this is one aspect of technology that shouldn't worry us. Professor Clare Wood, psychologist at the University of Coventry said, 'We are now starting to see consistent evidence that children's use of text-message abbreviations has a positive impact on their spelling skills. There is no evidence that children's language play when using mobile phones is damaging literacy development.'

- In a survey by the *Times Educational Supplement* and the charity e-Learning Foundation, more than half of teachers believe that children with no internet access are seriously disadvantaged in their education. Also, a fifth of the 585 teachers surveyed said internet access was essential for pupils' homework.

- Researchers at the University of London found that children who watched three or more hours of television a day were three months ahead of their peers who watched less than an hour a day, comforting parents who feel guilty about their reliance on the 'electronic nanny'. The report's lead author, Dr Alice Sullivan, senior academic at the university's Institute of Education, said the educational value of children's television had been 'underestimated', adding, 'It may also help expose some children to a broader vocabulary than they get at home.'

- A new study into the effects of computer games has revealed that fast-paced action games turn us into faster and better decision-makers. Scientists at the University of Rochester in New York tested a group of 18–25 year olds who were not normally video-gamers and discovered that after 50 hours of playing, those who played action-packed games such as Call of Duty made decisions 25 per cent faster than those who played more sedate games such as The Sims.

5:2

YOUR RELATIONSHIP

LIFE BEFORE MY 5:2 RELATIONSHIP FIX

It's 8.45 p.m. on a Saturday night and the children are settling down with us on the sofa to watch a family film. Bedtime is on the distant horizon, and I can't help wondering what happened to those endless evenings before children, or even when they were babies and sleeping soundly by suppertime.

We delight in having our children around, sharing the things we love doing with them, but the older they are, the more difficult it is for my husband and me to enjoy time together, just the two of us. Because we have been happy to let our kids colonise our company with the military efficiency of an army: advancing on small continents of time that we used to cherish – any serious, or gossipy, 'grown-up' conversation that they used to ignore as smaller children is now monitored, challenged, interrupted. They want to be part of it too, and are quick to pick up on exchanges that don't involve them: 'I can hear what you're talking to Dad about'; 'What are you saying about our Auntie's memory?'; 'Why are you talking about Alps climbers?'; 'Why are you whispering?'

I look at a pile of DVDs gathering dust on our mantelpiece for Saturday viewing – that first series of a TV show that my husband was going to watch all over again, to share it with me, a 1980s thriller we promised to see one evening. It hasn't happened. During the week, our children are in bed by 8.30 p.m., but the bulk of our weekend evenings is occupied territory.

Together for the last twenty years and married for the last nine, our relationship is strong. We enjoy each other's company, our friendship. If only there was more time. It takes energy to plan ahead and factor in spontaneity, something that is often lost in the struggle of domestic routine. Trips to Paris, Blackpool, even that pub around the corner, seem increasingly distant. Having a third child a little late has made it more difficult to spend the odd night alone. Most 44-year-old parents we know are, finally, off to the pub by themselves again, going to the odd music festival or having a weekend away. Instead, we are reliving the joys of night feeds, sterilising and dawn viewings of *Pingu*.

Of course, it is not only beleaguered parents who fail to carve out 'couple time'. Ben and Anna have been together since their teens – they grew up together in a small town and married in their late twenties. Ben runs his own PR business and Anna is an events manager. 'I can't remember the last time we went out as a couple,' says Anna. 'Because we met when we were young, we were always determined to be independent, even though we were a couple. We fell in love but never wanted to miss out on our single friends' lifestyle – going on holiday with them, and always going out with our separate groups of mates.' Now in their early thirties, their friends are in couples too, but the habit of socialising with other people more than with one another has stuck. 'As we both get busier in our jobs – Ben travels a lot with his work and I have to work a lot of evenings – we can go for days without seeing each other. We've become experts at keeping in touch on the hoof – FaceTime, text and emails – but it's something I'm becoming more aware of. We're getting married next year, and I'm starting to think if it's difficult getting time alone now, what will happen when we start a family?'

Ben and Anna have a strong foundation and are looking forward to getting married, but they need to somehow find a way to connect more with one another before they have children.

In our case, as in so many relationships, I knew the key would be to focus on ring-fencing time for one another – making it happen, whatever the other distractions.

MAKING THE 5:2 CONNECTION

I began to make the relationship link to the principles of 5:2. Why not a moderate approach that looks to make good relationships better – nothing too seismic or scary – that would fit the easy compromise of the 5:2 ratio? Just like the 5:2 diet, a two-day relationship focus wouldn't be too full on, so would be ideal for couples that are essentially happy with one another but could also benefit from some part-time reflection, and some auditing and tweaking of their relationship habits.

I approached psychotherapist and author of *How to Stay Sane*, Philippa Perry, who immediately warmed to the idea and offers her advice on my seven steps for making the 5:2 relationship fix work for you. 'Focusing on your relationship for two days a week is achievable,' she says. 'When we're trying for change we often go for unrealistic goals that are bound to result in failure. Extreme action often leads to polarised behaviour which isn't good for our wellbeing and sanity. You don't have to think about it all the time. It offers a structure but not too much – it's down the line; in the middle, which is a good thing.'

Couple psychotherapist Professor Janet Reibstein, and author of *The Best-Kept Secret – How Love Can Last For Ever*, could also see the benefits. 'If you have two really good days of relating, you can help to ensure positive times together for you to think about in the other five. It also gives you a good space to redress issues that can build up over a week.'

For *The Best-Kept Secret*, Reibstein conducted over two hundred in-depth interviews with couples in order to investigate the formulas for their long-lasting marriages. For a two-day relationship focus, I too felt it was important to examine what can make a relationship flourish, rather than scrutinising the negatives. Studying what makes happy couples tick is a good place to start.

In Tolstoy's famous opening lines of his novel *Anna Karenina* we are told that 'Happy families are all alike; every unhappy family is unhappy in its own way', and it's this unifying 'alikeness' in happiness that grips many couple therapists, including one of the best known of them all, John Gottman, psychology professor and couple therapist who has predicted with 90 per cent accuracy which couples will divorce within six years.

In his and Nan Silver's book *The Seven Principles for Making Marriages Work*, Gottman says, 'I was not able to crack the code to saving marriages until I started to analyse what went right in happy marriages. After intensely studying happily married couples for as long as sixteen years, I now know that the key to reviving or divorce-proofing a relationship is not how you handle disagreements but in how you are with each other when you're not fighting.'

That is why the 5:2 approach here isn't aimed at relationships in crisis but focuses on strengthening and enhancing the positives.

THE 5:2 RELATIONSHIP FIX; aims and benefits

- A simple and feasible way of building friendship into your relationship twice a week.

- Flexible exercises that weave into your daily life and challenge old routines.

You and your partner will:

- Feel happier, able to engage in new, shared experiences and appreciate your life together more.

- Feel more able to talk, and to listen to one another, in a nonjudgemental way.

- Learn to appreciate shared memories and draw on a shared past – one of the most effective ways of strengthening any relationship.

- Feel confident and comfortable talking about your sex life and asking for what you want.

- Recognise the importance of the small details in your relationship.

GETTING STARTED ON THE 5:2 RELATIONSHIP FIX

Now you've read about my experience, and Ben and Anna's, and why 5:2 is the perfect ratio for a relationship boost, here's how to do it. These seven steps will outline a combination of techniques, exercises and reflections. Mix and match them how you please over your two-day relationship focus, and return to them once a fortnight.

SEVEN STEPS TO MAKE THE 5:2 RELATIONSHIP FIX WORK FOR YOU

1 Do a 'shared time' audit

Unless you are in the first giddy weeks of a new relationship, chances are you don't spend as much quality time with your partner as you'd like to or should, but even the most recent of romances can benefit from these seven-step exercises – designed to enhance any relationship.

The average couple spends two-and-a-half hours a day in each other's company, although much of that is watching TV, or on different screens but in the same room. Time together in the home increases when you become parents, but it also becomes much less exclusive – suddenly your relationship is shared with smaller members of the household.

Whatever your relationship stage, this is a valuable way of quantifying exactly how much time you share and engage with one another. Time alone together isn't an indulgence, as you'll learn here, but a crucial resource; memories and positive associations protect your relationship when harder times strike. An hour here or there that you enjoy alone together during your two relationship days will build resilience for the rest of the week when you have less time to focus on your partner.

Sit down together with a pen and paper. Spend fifteen minutes or so thinking about the last week or two, or even earlier, and make a list of those times when you really paid attention to each other, felt listened to or understood by your partner. Whatever the context, however mundane or momentary, profound or memorable, it doesn't really matter: laughing at your partner's recollection of an embarrassing moment while you brush your teeth, a night out alone or a walk together, an engaging discussion in your local supermarket or preparing a weekday meal together.

As Reibstein says, 'One of the main findings from my research is that couples don't make enough time for each other – you may not think this is the case unless you do this exercise. When I do this in therapy and they go back over their week, they're astonished at how few hours they actually spend in each other's company, in a meaningful way.'

Once you've written your lists, compare them with one another and discuss some of those memories you've written down. Are there any surprises in there? Have you chosen the same examples? Can you even remember the times your partner has mentioned and is it a pleasant reminder? Are you annoyed that they have forgotten a moment that's crystal clear for you? This exercise can be returned to every fortnight or so, as a way of checking in and reminding each other of shared times and why you enjoyed them.

Here's how my list looked:

- Waking early and chatting, often about something on the radio, for ten minutes or so before our youngest wakes and the mayhem of a morning routine takes over.

- Unexpectedly being in a car alone for twenty minutes, without arguing children and a shrieking toddler, on a drive to pick up friends. 'Wow, we're alone in the car, it's spooky,' I remember saying.

- Chatting to my husband while we prepare – or rather he prepares – the evening meal (more on how he feels about that in Step 3).

- Having a glass of wine together in the evening (though not on Drink Diet days, of course) – a pleasant ritual that cements the moment when we stop work and discuss the day.

- Last real shared time away from children? That would be my husband's birthday six months earlier – a one-hour run together in the morning followed by lunch and the cinema.

His list looked a bit like this:

- A friend's birthday meal where, by accident, we were seated next to each other and chatted for a lot of the evening.

- Sending one another frequent emails of stuff that's caught our interest: serious, trivial, often silly.

- Waking early and discussing what's on the news.

- Ongoing discussion of a book that one of us has finished first. Does this count as shared activity? Probably not.

So the lists made the point: we clearly don't spend enough time together. The upside, we agreed, is that we are quite adept these days at catching up and connecting on the go, in the moment. Talking throughout each morning and evening, emailing and texting, while batting away interruptions from small children. 'Eating together, going to bed at the same time – a certain amount of that has to happen,' says Reibstein. And it does in our household; it gets us through, but it's no substitute for a date night.

I didn't realise the impact sharing certain routine tasks has in a relationship, until I was doing this exercise and comparing my current relationship with my last one. I always go to bed at the same time as my partner and often we'll read in bed. It's part of a ritual where I'll bring up a glass of water for both of us and he'll make us tea in the morning.

Somehow we feel in the same zone, where we're not consciously thinking about it but we're doing little things to make the other feel better. In my last relationship, we'd often watch TV in different rooms and I'd usually go up to bed first – now I can see that was the first symptom of us feeling distant, unconnected to each other.

Kim, 32

I started to go and greet my partner in the hall when I heard his key in the door. OK, so it's a little "1950s housewife" but it meant that we actually engaged with each other and kissed hello instead of just glancing up whilst loading the dishwasher like usual.

Caroline, 43

② Make a date

This isn't a demand to dress up and sit in an overpriced restaurant, or even to leave the house. It is, however, crucial to carve in stone when you can spend two hours alone every week, the two of you, engaging in something more than watching a DVD box set. It could be eating a meal together, having a pint, a game of tennis or Scrabble, or just a chat – exclusive time when phones are switched off and no one else is around.

'You do need to set aside couple time, but don't be prescriptive,' says Philippa Perry. 'I don't like the excuse "we can't afford date night" – do something that doesn't involve money. Go for a long walk each week with your partner, which is what I do every weekend. It can be much better than going for a drink because there's less pressure.' Walking together helps you to reflect, discuss, make important decisions. When President Obama is dwelling on a course of action, does he immediately call a meeting in the White House? No, he goes for a walk with his chief of staff.

'You're not facing each other while you walk so it's less intense and the odd silence doesn't matter. You're relaxed too because of the endorphins from the exercise. I love the ritual of it,' says Perry.

Whatever activity you decide upon, make it a sanctuary and, yes, even better if you can factor in sex too. Susanna Abse, director of the Tavistock Centre for Couple Relationships, says, 'If you know that time is yours and you don't have to ask for it, then you're avoiding the possibility of rejection, getting slighted or hurt. It's a containing routine where you can give one another your full attention and, if you want to, go beyond that.'

Walk your way to a happy relationship

'We've been married for thirty-seven years and you think, "What on earth would we talk about if we did something together?" But our weekly four-hour walk around London is so satisfying. We factor in our own little rituals, including a visit to a real-ale pub at the end. It's one of the few situations I can think of where you're alone with one another uninterrupted for so long but there's very little pressure. If you don't talk, it doesn't matter – that feels very important to both of us. Or you can cast thoughts out into the air in a freer way, rather than aiming an arrow at one person, and the other person may respond but doesn't have to. Then there's the constant change of scenery that you can comment on, or where you're going to have lunch. You can often find yourself enjoying deep discussions too. It feels as if you can go in lots of different ways, and it's an activity that takes you out of the clutches of domestic routine. You always feel in a better frame of mind once you've both started out. It's a good conversational point too – between ourselves, but socially too. People are always impressed when I turn down an engagement and say, "No, I couldn't do that, I'm out walking with my husband."'

Pauline, 55

Every relationship expert would place time together high on their list as the cornerstone of any thriving relationship, and it's something that you should schedule in immediately on one of your two relationship days.

'All the successful couples I spoke to do this,' says Reibstein. 'One couple had six children but always made it to their local pub each week, throughout their lives, and that's why they were able to carry on enjoying each other.'

If expense or leaving the house is an issue, as it is with me, schedule an evening at home – it might take more commitment but it can work. 'You need to say "This is our time" to your children,' says Reibstein. 'Stand up to them; you have to let your children know that you're giving that seriousness to your own relationship. If you can't put yourselves first sometimes, it is the slow death of a relationship.'

> *One way we really enjoy a window of time is getting the train to work twice a week. After doing this step, I decided to commit to getting up earlier for two days so we could have that hour to share with no one else to distract us.*
>
> *We've been doing it for a month now and it's such a nice way of catching up, talking about what's in the papers, what we're doing at the weekend. We'll often find ourselves having an entire conversation about a holiday we've been on. "Do you remember that place we visited?" etc. When you're in the nine-to-five slog, it's good to reminisce about fun things you've done. It's not deep, demanding conversation but it feels like a daily connection that I really appreciate.*
>
> Anna, 28

Make a date with yourself

During your two-day relationship focus, think about ways, especially if you have children, of allowing your partner small freedoms from the coalface of domesticity. Let them have time for themselves: an hour for a coffee, an afternoon off for shopping, or a day-trip with friends while you look after the children. They'll be appreciative and much more willing to give you time away in return.

> *I negotiate with my wife to let me go on cycling weekends away for a night or two every three months or so. I love the escape and the adventure, to reflect on all my relationships*

when I'm away. I find it makes me so much more appreciative, of my wife letting me do it and what I'm coming home to. Those last few hours cycling home, all I want to do is get back to my wife and children.

Matthew, 40

Every weekend was taken up with our own hobbies – he'd go mountain-biking, I'd play tennis. So I persuaded him to try tennis and I joined him on his bike ride. I wouldn't say we now do it every weekend, but I enjoyed it and got to see why he loves it so much, which helped me not feel so rejected when he goes off for hours on end. We've also taking to going to the cinema instead of watching telly – taking turns to pick the film. Yes, we're still staring at a screen in silence, but it feels like quality time and we chat about the film afterwards.

Nicky, 30

3 **Build empathy**

Empathy lies at the heart of any romantic or committed relationship. According to Reibstein, it was the key virtue that all her happily married couples shared. 'Couples that could solve a conflict managed to see beyond it. They knew that tending to wounded feelings and making amends was as important, more so than what they were arguing about.'

One key exercise that is designed specifically to improve you and your partner's empathy skills is reflective listening – it doesn't take long and can easily fit into one of your 5:2 relationship days. It is also a skill that can be substantially improved by practising once a week, as long as you stick to the simple guidelines.

191

Letting your partner talk for three minutes about any issue that's on their mind and then reflecting back their thoughts and feelings is a powerful way of immediately viewing life from their perspective and of increasing tolerance and understanding. All you need is fifteen minutes and a quiet space to sit together. Start with fairly neutral feelings and reflections, while you're mastering the process. Each week you can build up to more intimate and honest reflections, as you begin to feel safe and confident in talking and being listened to.

'It can very usefully become, on your two focused relationship days, a half-hour window to share something that you may not normally get the chance to do throughout the rest of the week. It's about finding out what you're really thinking and feeling rather than working on assumptions,' says Perry.

Here's how:

1) One partner talks, describing a simple event that may or may not have involved their partner and how it made them feel.

2) The listener must concentrate fully and cannot interrupt while their partner talks – they must be allowed to speak freely.

3) The listener should then become the speaker and summarise their partner's thoughts and feelings in their own words whilst mirroring as much as possible the feelings and nonverbal communications of their partner, i.e. their tone of voice, posture, manner. Don't digress and make assumptions of your own, stick exactly to their main points. To help you reflect back, you can begin sentences with:
'So what you feel is ... '
'You're wondering if ... '
'It sounds to me like you ... '

4) Switch roles for another five or so minutes and then discuss how it felt from each perspective. Did it challenge any assumptions? What surprised you? Is there any behaviour you'd change as a result?

Our listening exercise sounded like this:

> Husband: 'Er, I seem to be doing nearly all the cooking in the evenings at the moment. I really enjoy cooking but I'd really like it if you cooked the odd meal as a treat, a nice thing to do for me. I'd really appreciate it.'

I repeat it back to him, mirroring his actions, tone of voice, etc., while he nods.

> My go: 'I feel that you do a lot of the cooking because I always have to put our 2-year-old to bed, change her nappy, bathe her and, I guess, I do sometimes feel it's one-sided.'

> Husband: 'Ah, but the reason that happens is … '

A brief derailment when I remind him he's not supposed to express an opinion, only reflect what I'm saying – which can be trickier than it sounds.

As we repeated our scenarios, something interesting happened for both us that I wouldn't necessarily have guessed at looking at the simple series of steps. Even our brief five-minute exchange was surprisingly powerful; we chose a subject that crops up frequently but this time we felt we were able to handle it much more constructively, taking time to make the other one feel heard rather than leaping to the defence. For the first time, we both agreed that once a week I will cook the evening meal while my husband does the night routine with our youngest. The exercise doesn't advise that you agree on a solution but, if the reflective listening works well, it feels like a natural next step to discuss a compromise, a way of moving forward.

> *I tried active listening with my partner when she came home from work, frazzled and down about a work crisis. Just sitting on the sofa, echoing back what she was talking about helped her so much more than making sympathetic noises with half an eye on the TV, which is my usual strategy. It felt strange not to make suggestions or offer solutions – although I now realise trying to "fix" a problem isn't always what she wants. It turns out just being heard and supported was a big comfort.*
>
> Jon, 40

4 Get to know each other

This exercise, from John Gottman and Nan Silver's *The Seven Principles for Making Marriages Work*, has got to be one of the most enjoyable tests you can do with your partner, which manages to serve a greater purpose too. Gottman says, 'Getting to know your spouse better is an ongoing process. In fact it's a life process. So expect to return to this exercise to update your knowledge about one another. Happy couples don't magically "know" one another.' They are continually curious, communicative and never assume to know what their partner is thinking; they ask.

When you first play, overlook any initial lapses in knowledge ('So you really don't know where I was born?') and approach it with humour and a glass of wine. The more you try this, the more you will learn – playing once a fortnight would be ideal. This gives you the opportunity to win your partner's admiration ('You remembered my favourite Robert de Niro film!') and express some gratitude of your own ('Ah, you really think I look sexy wearing that?').

Sit down together with a pen and paper. Both write down your answers and then take it in turns to read them out. If your partner answers correctly (it's up to you to judge), he or she receives the number of points next to the question. If they answer incorrectly, they get no points. The winner is the person with the most points after you've both answered the questions, although the game shouldn't be viewed so much as a competition but a *Mr & Mrs* style quiz to open up discussion.

1) Name my closest friends or friend. (2)

2) What's my favourite pop group or composer? (2)

3) What was I wearing when we first met? (2)

4) Where was I born? (1)

5) What stresses am I facing at the moment? (2)

6) What is my favourite unfulfilled dream? (4)

7) When do I most like to have sex? (3)

8) What was one of my best childhood experiences? (2)

9) What do I like most to do with my time off? (2)

10) What is my favourite film? (2)

11) What do I fear most? (4)

12) Which side of the bed do I prefer? (1)

13) What medical problems do I worry about most? (2)

14) What is my favourite romantic restaurant? (2)

15) Name one of my favourite novels. (2)

16) Name two of the people I admire most. (4)

17) What is my favourite sex position? (3)

18) What spot on my body is most sensitive? (4)

19) What was my most embarrassing moment? (3)

20) What is my favourite outfit to wear when I want to look sexy? (3)

21) Do I prefer flowers or chocolates? (2)

22) What is my favourite holiday? (2)

23) What physical quality am I most attracted to in the opposite sex? (3)

24) When was the first time I had sex? (2)

25) What's my favorite TV programme? (3)

26) What is the date of our anniversary? (1)

27) What did I think about you when we first met? (4)

28) When did we have our first kiss? (1)

29) What is my favorite getaway place? (3)

30) What am I most sad about? (3)

Notes to self

Entertaining and we'll definitely try it again – and add in a few questions of our own too. There were a few surprises; my husband was touched that I remembered with clarity his happiest childhood memory, as well as his most embarrassing moment at school. I'm still piqued he thinks that one of the people I most admire today is Kate Moss, not Sylvia Plath or Tina Fey, but it created animated discussion, and a positive feeling about our shared knowledge.

> *This exercise made us both smile and it was nice to have an excuse to turn the telly off and do something together. I also appreciated how much my partner knows about me and felt a little bit guilty I didn't know nearly as much about him! I'm not a very good listener and it really reminded me that it's something I should work at – I find I'm asking more sneaky questions about his past now so I can impress him when we play again in two weeks' time.*
>
> Ruth, 26

5 Draw on the past

Your knowledge of one another is, in fact, your greatest resource, which is why Step 4 is devoted to building it up, like a *Mastermind* specialist subject, week by week. This step builds on those memories, encouraging you to remember and appreciate your partner's positive traits.

Couples who have the best chance of happiness are those who can tap into these good memories in times of conflict, to maintain a sense of perspective. As in, 'He or she is so self-absorbed, critical, unaffectionate, etc. at the moment but they're not always like this. Remember that time last month when he or she did this for me.'

This was another key finding in Reibstein's research. 'Couples who thrived could hold on to the idea that the relationship wasn't just a sum of the bad times. They were more able to look back and access a sense of happier moments, basically remembering what was pleasurable about being together.' And these couples are more able to replenish that store cupboard of positive memories as they go along.

This dynamic, Reibstein discovered, was an unconscious habit; they hadn't been in therapy. But, as she says, it's a skill that can be learnt and which can soon become a habit.

Gottman, too, places great importance on the link between a couple's fondness and admiration for one another, and an ability to draw on their past for succour. 'By simply reminding yourself of your partner's positive qualities, even as you grapple with each other's flaws, you can prevent a happy relationship from deteriorating.'

Here's how, with his 'appreciation' exercise, taken from his book, co-authored with Nan Silver, *The Seven Principles for Making Marriages Work*.

From the list below, choose three items that you think are characteristic of your partner. If there are more than three, still circle just three (you can choose another three if you decide to do this exercise again). Even if you can recall only one instance when your partner displayed this characteristic, you can circle it.

Loving, Sensitive, Perceptive, Intelligent, Thoughtful, Generous, Loyal, Truthful, Strong, Energetic, Sexy, Decisive, Creative, Imaginative, Fun, Attractive, Interesting, Supportive, Funny, Considerate, Affectionate, Organised, Resourceful, Fit, Cheerful, Coordinated, Graceful, Elegant, Gracious, Playful, Caring, A great friend, Exciting, Full of plans, Shy, Vulnerable, Committed, Involved, Expressive, Active, Careful, Reserved, Adventurous, Receptive, Reliable, Responsible, Dependable, Nurturing, Warm, Virile, Kind, Gentle, Practical, Humorous, Witty, Relaxed, Beautiful, Handsome, Rich, Calm, Lively, A great partner, A great parent, Assertive, Protective, Tender, Powerful, Flexible, Understanding, Silly.

For each item you chose, briefly think of an actual incident that illustrates this characteristic of your partner. Write it down as follows:

1) Characteristic _____

   Incident: _____

2) Characteristic _____

   Incident: _____

3) Characteristic _____

   Incident: _____

You can approach the exercise in a light-hearted way but it helps if it's in the spirit of being genuine and sincere too. Share your answers, comparing your thoughts and letting one another know why you value these traits so highly.

'Couples who began the session sitting stiffly and awkwardly suddenly seem relaxed. Looking at them, you can tell that something they had lost has been regained,' says Gottman.

Dan's illness has been dragging on for weeks and it has taken its toll on our relationship – he's been negative, moany and self-pitying, not three characteristics I should remember him for. So I tried the exercise and it reminded me of how he is normally – upbeat, enthusiastic and caring. It has helped me cope and reminded me it's only temporary. It also made me realise how hard it is for him and we had a good chat about it and planned a holiday when he's better.
   Chloe, 32

Sex matters

One emotion that erodes a couple's sex life more than any other is brooding resentment, often unconscious. 'You may not have a strong awareness of it on the surface but underneath you may carry a sense of irritation or unfairness,' says psychologist and sex therapist Pamela Stephenson Connolly. 'These types of feelings really affect desire. You don't want to even touch someone who is making you mad on some level.'

She advises clients in this situation to try one simple exercise twice a week. It's a three-part spoken statement with the following prompts: 'I feel … '; 'Because … '; 'I would appreciate it if you … ' and each partner should take it in turns to fill in those blanks.

It's a very nonthreatening way of expressing a frustration and asking for change. 'If you can sit down and do this twice weekly, issues will come up and you'll become so much more aware of feelings you're harbouring and they become aired.'

One you've built up confidence, you can begin to use this exercise to broach sexual desires too. 'This is a great way to make a sensual request,' says Stephenson Connolly. '"I really enjoy making love with you but I wonder if … " All sexual relationships need to have a tune-up, not because things aren't going well, but your desires can change from week to week. There can be many reasons – from hormonal cycles to fatigue – why sexual needs change, and this is a safe, nonjudgemental way of reminding a partner that may be something a little bit different is needed.'

We've been going out for a year and, from the start, initiating sex has always been down to me. It's something I've become more aware of as we've fallen into more of a routine and I'm maybe a bit frustrated about – I've just been embarrassed about how to broach it. I've worried that maybe she doesn't desire me or is she just shy? I wanted to talk about it without looking critical or resentful so when it came to my turn, I said, "I feel the pressure is on me to initiate sex. Because you never start it and that can sometimes make me wonder if you want sex as much as me. I'd really appreciate it if once in a while you could make the first move."

We felt self-conscious at first but she was totally reassuring. Even admitting it to her made me feel so much better and now I'm sure something will change.

Mark, 32

We have been together for ten years and I had noticed that we had stopped having oral sex. At first we used to, but that was during the honeymoon stage when we were trying to impress each other. My partner has never been very interested in it and never initiates it. But I love it and it was a major part of previous relationships. So I suggested we have a bath together, and that afterwards we try it. She was more open to it and it brought a new element back into our love life. Having a bath together was a lovely sensual experience and helped us break out of our sexual rut. It's excruciating talking about sex and we both avoid it for fear of rejection or looking silly, but approaching it in this relaxed way made it easier.

Tim, 37

'It's starting to take responsibility for setting the scene sexually, about the when and the where of a sexual encounter,' say Stephenson Connolly. 'It's good to realise these kinds of things can change.'

7 Focus on the small things

Pay attention to the smaller details, even twice a week, and the benefits will be disproportionate. Four years ago, Sir David Brailsford, performance director for British Cycling and general manager of Team Sky, explained his winning philosophy, the 'aggregation of marginal gains', as searching for the 1 per cent margin for improvement in every area of your life. Brailsford's team would focus on this idea: from the cycle mechanics and beyond, no detail was too small to improve upon. So the team were given lessons in how to wash their hands to minimalise their risk of illness. A team chef would keep an eye on the kitchen where they stayed to reduce any chance of food poisoning. Trainers made sure the bedding was hypoallergenic and a psychologist was on hand to help the cyclists.

Inevitably Brailsfords's marginal gains principle has already been applied to other areas of life, including business and education, but its relevance for couple relationships is just as key – raising the bar on seemingly trivial aspects of daily behaviour for maximum benefit.

Here's how to apply marginal gains to your relationship:

Sit down together with a pen and paper. Both make a list of the smallest everyday actions and kindnesses that you think would make your partner happier. Aim for four or more.

Be as specific as you can. It could be improving an existing behaviour – 'Rather than leaving the towel on the floor, I'll put it back' – or introducing something new. 'I'll bring you a cup of tea each morning which you always do for me.'

You may be surprised that your partner doesn't want you to do a certain thing for them. 'This isn't about being right,' says Harriet Drake, couple psychotherapist at the Tavistock Centre for Couple Relationships, who often uses this exercise. 'What's interesting is that partners can get it wrong about what they think their partner may want but it gets a discussion going about what you really would appreciate, and what doesn't matter to you at all. There may be genuine shocks, like "When did you stop liking that?" or "I didn't know you even liked that?"'

Now you've got a more accurate sense of those tiny details that please your partner, write them down on slips of paper (four each is fine), fold them up and put them in a bowl. 'These are things you can do for your partner over two days of each week,' says Drake. Choose a new one each time.

> *Previously, making requests to my partner, such as asking him not to dry towels on the radiator (as they get rust marks) made him feel criticised, defensive and angry, but when it became a mutual discussion where we could both voice our irritations it defused the situation. He had been choosing not to comment about things that niggled him because he didn't want to cause upset, but once he did I felt happy to oblige and now stack the dishwasher his way – it's a compromise we're both happy about.*
> Nina, 42

COMMON QUESTIONS

Which two days should I choose to focus on my relationship?

Choose nonconsecutive days and, ideally, one at the weekend when you can go out together. Don't focus on the exercises for more than forty minutes on any one day and, as Philippa Perry advises, no discussions about anything serious after 10 p.m.

What should I bear in mind for the other five days?

Whatever you learn and enjoy in your two-day focus will permeate the other days and you'll naturally want to behave a bit better once you can feel the benefits, rather like on the 5:2 diet. Don't overthink your relationship or feel you have to introduce what you've learnt into every exchange and communication. Perry says, 'On the 5:2 diet you're cutting your calories down by 20 per cent, it's not dramatic – this shouldn't be either. Don't get too obsessive about it.'

'Enjoying some time apart – an hour or two here or an evening there – for the rest of the week is really beneficial too,' says Perry. 'For those days, really try to live your own life as well, especially if you're a couple who tend to do everything together. So when you focus on those two relationship days, you've got something to bring back to them.'

Which other 5:2 life areas combine well with relationships?

Try combining your 5:2 **Relationship** days with 5:2 Your **Fitness** – sharing a run or a walk together. It's also a natural complement to your 5:2 **Screen** diet: use the time you might have spent on your laptop, iPad or phone working through the 5:2 relationship steps or enjoying a night out.

If you are on the 5:2 diet then perhaps best to avoid combining with this one. As journalist Tim Dowling discovered when he tested out the 5:2 relationship fix while his wife was fasting. 'One of the advantages of the 5:2 diet is you can choose your fasting days, and my wife often swaps them around. More than once I come down to lunch with a compliment in mind to find her hunched over a mean-looking salad.' Use different days to avoid any friction and stick to the ones you've chosen to avoid overlap.

RELATIONSHIP FACTS

- According to John Gottman, there are four negative behaviours that are the doom of any relationship, otherwise known as 'The Four Horsemen of the Apocalypse':

  1) Criticism: stating one's complaints as a defect in one's partner's personality, i.e. giving the partner negative trait attributions. Example: 'You always talk about yourself. You are so selfish.'

  2) Contempt: statements that come from a relative position of superiority. Contempt is the greatest predictor of divorce and must be eliminated. Example: 'You're an idiot.'

  3) Defensiveness: self-protection in the form of righteous indignation or innocent victimhood. Defensiveness wards off a perceived attack. Example: 'It's not my fault that we're always late; it's your fault.'

  4) Stonewalling: emotional withdrawal from interaction. Example: The listener does not give the speaker the usual nonverbal signals that the listener is 'tracking' the speaker and concentrating on what they are saying.

- Partners who behave towards one another in these ways are much more likely to be divorced – an average of 5.6 years after the wedding. Emotional withdrawal and anger are predictive factors in later instances of divorce: an average of 16.2 years after the wedding.

- A healthy partnership requires a balanced level of positive and negative interaction – Gottman suggests that a ratio of

5 positive to 1 negative – during conflict discussions – will enable a relationship to thrive. Again, don't go overboard on trying to improve your positive–negative ratio throughout the week – be aware in a neutral rather than self-critical way.

- Couples who are realistic about one another's faults are easily the happiest, particularly the ones that are able to tolerate difference and diversity in their relationship. 'Couples spend year after year trying to change each other's minds, but it can't be done,' says Gottman. 'This is because most of their disagreements are rooted in fundamental differences of lifestyle, personality or values.'

- Being married makes you healthier and live longer. *The State of the Nation Report* (2006) found that on average married people have better physical health and longevity than those who never married. In men, the mortality rate is 250 per cent higher in unmarried men than in married men, compared to 50 per cent higher in unmarried women.

- Although many see it as cementing a relationship, having a baby can cause serious problems. According to a study by relationship charity OnePlusOne, two-thirds of couples felt worried about aspects of their relationship after becoming parents. 40 per cent of new mothers were worried that they were no longer sexually attractive to their partner and a quarter of fathers felt concerned that their partner's sex drive had dipped.

- Tenderness from your partner can help you cope in stressful situations. A study by the University of North Carolina discovered that ten minutes of holding hands followed by a twenty-second hug reduced the blood pressure and heart rate of participants when they were in fraught situations, such as public speaking.

- Regular sex boosts your immune system, according to researchers at Wilkes University in Pennsylvania. People who have sex once or twice a week produce 30 per cent more immunoglobulin A, an important illness-fighting substance.

5:2

YOUR
WORRY

LIFE BEFORE MY 5:2 WORRY DIET

Ever since I can remember, worry has been a familiar companion, never far away. Small intrusive thoughts worm their way into my psyche from one minute to the next. By nature I speculate, analyse and interpret – good if you're a journalist, but not so great when it seeps into your everyday life, creating a spiral of endless fretting. Snippy barbed anxieties scroll through my consciousness, usually in an endless loop of self-questioning – when you see my worry list in Step 1, you'll see what I mean.

Vivid images unfurl, like snippets from trashy made-for-TV movies, giving each groundless anxiety more volume and power. When one of my children says they feel they're unwell before we're due to fly abroad for our summer holiday, which they're prone to do, I'm hard-wired to fast-forward in a calamitous way – I visualise my child, feverish, in a foreign hospital bed, miles from home, and think how much less stressful it would be to stay at home. If my 11-year-old son walks to the corner shop, for a fleeting second a newspaper headline will dart through my mind: 'Last time I ever saw my son alive.'

These are flashes, thankfully, rather than full-blown anxieties that affect my day-to-day life. Often they are simply thoughts that come and then go, dramatic as they may seem, without engaging me, and then simply pass away. But, still, I'd rather live without them.

If this seems completely alien to you, then you're one of the fortunate ones who can skip back lightheartedly to the 5:2 Your Fitness or Productivity chapter. If, on the other hand, this all sounds ominously familiar, keep on reading – inevitably you'll have earmarked the 5:2 Your Drink and 5:2 Your Money chapters too, both familiar territory to the eternal worrier.

Rewind twenty years: my brush with anxiety

My husband, then boyfriend, is driving us through the Forest of Dean in his ancient Mini. Windows open, music loud, blasting through the English countryside. Not a worry on the horizon, only endless blue sky and gentle rolling hills. We are still young, six more years of freedom before mortgage and babies transform our lives. And yet ... I've been feeling strange all day; a sense of general unease has been nagging at the periphery. We were out late drinking in London the evening before and up early for our break. My stomach feels taut, my palms sweaty.

Then it happens. My boyfriend has to brake abruptly as another car passes us on a narrow lane. It's nothing too extreme. The car passes and we accelerate again. But that jolt is enough. My general unease shifts to nameless dread. My lips and fingertips begin to tingle and, strangely, that cobalt-blue sky has now taken on a menacing jaundiced tinge. I feel weirdly divorced from reality, watching myself from a distance. My throat tightens and each breath takes Herculean effort. 'I think you may have to pull over, I feel ... strange,' I manage to whisper.

By the time we stop further up the road, I feel much better, puzzled by what just happened, but definitely 'me' again. A bit of deep breathing, lots of water and an early night and I feel fine the next day, no more symptoms.

When I get home, I start to confide in friends about the experience and it's surprising, and reassuring, how many of them have been through something similar. Was it a full-blown anxiety attack? An end-of-twenties wobble, waking up to the fact that real responsibilities were looming on the horizon as my thirties approached? Or just one too many gin-and-tonics and not enough sleep? I'll never really know because it only happened once, thankfully. What it actually turned out to be was a timely wake-up call, my body signalling to me in no uncertain terms that I should drink a little less and exercise a little more – which I've done pretty much ever since.

What really helped for a few weeks afterwards was one simple breathing exercise. I'd imagine my breath was a circle: visualise that circle in my head, inhale for half of it, for around four seconds, and exhale for the other, then repeat. I could practise it anywhere – in bed before I fell asleep, in a crowded Tube station, or walking down the street. For me that was a great comfort.

Keeping anxiety at bay

I would describe myself as a moderate worrier, able to cope, generally happy and sanguine. Still, I'd certainly like to be able to worry less – who wouldn't?

The older I get, the less likely this seems – as a parent, worry takes on a whole new dimension.

The usual suspects scatter my thoughts in all directions. Are the children eating healthily enough? How long before we're dragged into another war? I should visit my parents more, but when?

Reducing anxiety, most experts agree, depends ultimately upon understanding ourselves. If we can get to the root of who we are, and why, then calm contentment will be ours. There's just the small question of how.

For psychoanalyst Sigmund Freud and his followers, conscious thought was the tip of the iceberg: true understanding of the self lay in the unconscious and could be unlocked only with the help of a skilled practitioner. Psychoanalysis and psychotherapy continue to rely on the notion that our wellbeing depends on continually evaluating our past.

With positive psychology, however, there has been a significant shift in the last fifteen years or so, to the idea that self-awareness doesn't have to be a process of lengthy introspection. The notion that the solution to much of our discontent need not lie in the past forms the basis of cognitive behavioural therapy (CBT).

American psychologist Albert Ellis, seen by many as the father of cognitive behavioural techniques, believed much of our unhappiness arises from allowing our 'wants' to turn into 'musts' – as in 'I "must" be happy.' 'Pretty much every time a human being gets disturbed, they're sneaking in, consciously or unconsciously, a "must".' 'Musts' create too much pressure, increasing self-criticism when we feel we can't achieve them. We need to become more aware of our 'musts', so we can let them go. The emphasis is on changing the way we think in the here and now.

What I was looking for was a technique that could embrace all this as well as slot in neatly with the 5:2 ratio. I wanted a flexible antidote for mild worriers with the promise that focusing on anxiety twice a week could kick-start a long-term change in mindset.

That's when I remembered an interview I carried out four years ago for a piece about the psychology of happiness with Professor Mark Williams of Oxford University. At that point, he hadn't yet written his bestselling book, co-authored with Dr Danny Penman, *Mindfulness: A Practical Guide to Finding Peace in a Frantic World.* He was still developing the technique, along with his colleagues: Mindfulness-Based Cognitive Therapy (MBCT), a method that yields impressive results.

Central to Williams's approach is 'noticing' emotions and physical sensations, without reflection or analysis; simply 'seeing' your thoughts coming and going.

He suggests starting with the smaller details in life: training your poorly disciplined mind not to wander away from the present moment. 'If you're drinking a cup of tea, are you really enjoying that tea, or planning what you'll be doing in half an hour? The problem is, we tend to plan, and to grade life: "When I get home from the supermarket, then I can relax"; "When I go on holiday, that's when life is good"; "When I'm at work, that's when life isn't interesting." But these are all moments of your life you're not living. If we can be present right here and now, it's much more difficult to worry about the past or the present.'

Within eight weeks of following similar techniques, Professor Williams says, people start to notice for the first time how the mind is drawn into fretful cycles of 'what if?' scenarios, which mean we end up 'living more in our head than we do in our life'. In two research trials with people suffering recurring depressive episodes, Mindfulness-Based Cognitive Therapy halved the chances of depression returning.

As Oliver Burkeman observes in his book *The Antidote: Happiness for People Who Can't Stand Positive Thinking*, 'Sometimes the most valuable of all talents is to be able not to seek resolution; to notice the craving for completeness or certainty or comfort, and not feel compelled to follow where it leads.' And if you can practise this for a small amount each week, then so much the better.

MAKING THE 5:2 CONNECTION

Still on my 5:2 diet, I began to wonder if a selection of mindfulness meditation techniques could work well in a similar ratio. I liked the idea of something that didn't stray into New Age philosophy or the overly relentless optimism of much positive psychology.

Professor Williams was encouraging about the idea when I talked to him again. 'It's a way of saying two days a week I'm going to give it my best shot with longer exercises and what I learn from this will permeate the other five days. It's a healthy compromise for people who've either tried it before but feel guilty they can't do it seven days or week, or maybe they want a taster.'

I also talked to Dr Robert L. Leahy, director of the American Institute for Cognitive Therapy in New York and author of *The Worry Cure*. He says, 'The 5:2 approach is a good way of jump-starting habits that help to reduce worry and we know the more you practise good habits, the stronger they become.'

THE 5:2 WORRY DIET; aims and benefits

- The 5:2 Worry Diet can help you drastically reduce stress and anxiety by focusing on exercises for no more than thirty minutes, twice a week.

- It applies the principles of the 5:2 diet – focusing intensely twice a week to enable you to see life in a different way for the other five.

- Simple, straightforward exercises that can add dimension to everyday tasks, and help you to live in the moment.

- Focuses on your sleep 'hygiene' for your Worry Diet days only, to ensure a better night's rest *all* week.

- These techniques are also invaluable for many of the other 5:2 areas you may wish to focus on – in particular the Screen Life Diet, Drink Diet and Fitness Plan.

GETTING STARTED ON THE 5:2 WORRY DIET

Now you've read about my relationship with worry and why I decided to apply the 5:2 approach to reducing anxiety, here's how to make it work.

In this section, I'll be outlining mindfulness exercises and cognitive therapy techniques with the help of Professor Mark Williams and Dr Robert Leahy; a perfect combination from two of the leading experts in worry.

I will also be recommending ways of improving your sleep routine, with advice from psychologist and fatigue specialist Dr Paul Jackson. Poor-quality sleep is increasingly linked to a range of physiological and emotional problems. According to a recent study of nearly 40,000 UK employees, only 15 per cent said they felt revived by their sleep. Often it's a vicious cycle where stress is the trigger and then the lack of sleep makes anxiety feel much more acute. Dr Jackson suggests simple tips that can be practised twice a week and fit well with other 5:2 life areas – in particular 5:2 Your Drink, Screen Life and Fitness.

Along with my own experiences, as well as testimonies from other people who've tried them out, you can see how easily this approach can combat worry in a low-key but effective way.

Mix and match the breathing, meditation and written exercises outlined in Steps 2 to 5 – you're aiming for around thirty minutes for each Worry Diet day. Step 8 sets out exercises that fit into the rest of your week, but can fit neatly into your two-day worry fast too.

View the breathing exercises as the foundation of your two worry-free days. It's up to you how many you try, whatever feels comfortable. As they become more familiar to you, they may well fit naturally into your daily routine too. The mindfulness exercise in Step 3 is particularly good because it works with any daily activity, the more mundane the better.

SEVEN STEPS TO MAKE THE 5:2 WORRY DIET WORK FOR YOU

1 **Do a worry audit**

Like any diet, you need to quantify your habit, map out a realistic picture in order to track your progress. Getting your worries down in black and white will aid mindful reflection, and it can be a powerful way of reducing them too. Two years ago, research carried out among a group of students in Chicago showed that the simple act of making notes about their anxieties before taking an exam improved their performance by 20 per cent. The University of California also found that writing about an emotion was a way of calming down the brain and re-establishing mental balance.

Sit down with a notepad and pen and give yourself around fifteen minutes to reflect on and list your common worries and concerns, old and new, profound and trivial. Give as much or as little detail as you want. How frequently do you think about each problem? Is it a high-level, intense and all-encompassing worry or just a nagging sense of unease? Is there a particular time at which it strikes?

Here is what the list looked like for Russell, 46.

- I'm anxious about job security and about what I'd do if I lost my job. That goes hand-in-hand with worrying about not bringing enough money into the household. I also fret about whether my recently widowed mother is managing OK and not too lonely.

- On a daily basis I wonder how I'll ever fit all my work and home commitments in, about not spending enough time with my children. I continually worry I'm a slave to time, and I hate the idea I might miss out on something so I try to do it all. I need to edit my life in order to give myself more time which I guess is why I'm doing this.

My worry list began like this:

- Listened to an item on the *Today* programme about interest rates staying low for two years – felt relieved but it still triggered a persistent worry about when they finally increase. I wonder what even a 1 per cent increase would mean to our loan? This is a well-worn worry that bites around once a fortnight – I notice that even when it's a positive news item (interest rates are staying low for now), I 'hear' it as bad news ('So they're going to go up at some point, right?').

- Read an article about teenage boys and their exposure to online porn – triggers more general concern about the insidious effects of the internet on our children. A recent survey points to the fact they now read less than ever before, cause for yet more worry.

- I can't remember closing or locking the front door as I drive my daughter to art class. Should I explain my anxiety to my daughter, which I'm reluctant to do, or carry on with our journey? I tell my daughter in a breezy way that I have to check on something, drive back and the door is closed. On any journey I can be ambushed with this old perennial: did I turn off the gas ring? Did I switch off my hair straighteners?

- My parking permit is still outstanding. If I leave it another week, it will be out of date, yet I keep putting it off.

- That chicken I just gave to my 2-year-old was a day past its sell-by date. I thought it looked a bit grey, or was I imagining it?

It smelt OK but now I worry I should have thrown it away. A mild anxiety that crops up now and then when I've fed my children.

- What will it feel like when one of my parents dies? I would describe this as a background worry that remains but has become less intrusive as the years go by.

Hang on to your list, it will be invaluable for some of the other steps, in particular Dr Robert Leahy's worry exercises (see Step 5) where you'll be using these thoughts as your raw material.

Think about expanding your list into a regular journal where you can write and expand on your thoughts and concerns, updating it just twice a week on your Worry Diet days. According to recent research from the University of Minnesota, workers who kept a diary significantly lowered their stress levels. In a study by the University of California in 2009, brain scans of diarists showed they were less vulnerable to anxiety and that writing about their feelings helped them to reduce emotional upsets.

2 Focus on the breath

All mindfulness meditation returns to the crucial importance of the breath – how it helps to focus an anxious and distracted mind by bringing us back into the physical moment.

I've been doing these exercises for a few weeks now and I'm already starting to tune in to my breathing in times of stress to check my state of mind. If my stress levels are high, I know that, inevitably, my breathing will be more shallow, my chest more tense and constrained. As soon as I breathe slowly, deeply, methodically, the physical manifestation of that anxiety passes.

Clara, 35

The following meditation can be done twice a day on your two Worry Diet days and takes no longer than ten minutes. It also works well with the 'tensing and relaxing' exercise on the next page – you may want to try this one in the morning and the other in the evening.

1) Find a familiar space in your home where you know you won't be disturbed. Adjust your body until you feel comfortable. Experiment until you have found a posture that feels completely natural.

2) Close your eyes and bring awareness to your body by focusing on sensations of touch, what it feels like to be in contact with other surfaces – a chair, rug or mat.

3) Focus attention on the tops of your legs and work down to the feet and then the toes registering each physical sensation in the moment, however small and imperceptible it may feel.

4) Slowly move your focus up the body, through the ankles, the legs, then take a few moments for the torso (from the hips and bottom up to the shoulders, then left arm, right arm, wrists, hands, fingers). Finally notice the neck and the head; face, ears, scalp and hair.

5) Reflect for a minute or two on this awareness of the whole body, how little you probably pay attention to these sensations in the course of daily life, and how they make you feel.

6) Now focus on your breath as it moves in and out of your body at the abdomen. Aim for slower, longer, deeper breaths now – inhale for four seconds, hold for a couple of seconds and then exhale for four seconds.

When I try this exercise, my first realisation is how I only really tune into specific parts of my body when I'm feeling pain or, hopefully, pleasure! Paying close attention to the low-level humming of my body feels alien. I'm not sure what I should be listening for but, as I relax into it, I learn, as Professor Williams suggests, to be curious, opening myself up to the tiniest detail. 'How would I describe how the back of my heel feels on the carpet? What exactly is that sensation: burning, itching maybe?' It's a relief to focus on my body for a change rather than my endless thoughts.

'When you're noticing the body, be aware of the distinction between "thinking" about parts of your body and actually "feeling" what it is like from inside your body – which is what you should focus on,' says Professor Williams.

> *I find trying this exercise easier in the bath. I turn the light off and lie in the darkness, listening to the gentle ripples as my body floats around. I imagine being in the womb, where my whole experience is just about sensation.*
> Erica, 51

Tensing and relaxing

Follow the steps as above but now tense and relax every muscle group so the sensations are more noticeable.

As before, start with the feet and toes – tense and hold for three seconds – then let go and move up to the knees, thighs, bottom, arms, hands and fingers, neck, jaw, mouth and eyes. This is a rewarding exercise, I find, because it's satisfying to focus on that physical contrast between tensing up and letting go, to really notice something tangible, and it's also a relaxing sensation. For extra focus, breathe through the nose, hold for five seconds while the muscles tense, then exhale through the mouth on release.

3 Improve your sleep

When you sleep well, your body and mind can relax; you feel rejuvenated and more resilient when you wake up in the morning and, of course, a lot less anxious.

Dr Paul Jackson suggests bearing the following in mind just twice a week to boost overall sleep hygiene:

- No drink. 'Even one glass of wine within a couple of hours of bedtime will disrupt sleep "architecture",' says Dr Jackson. 'When you sleep you progress through different stages. One and Two is light sleep, Three is deeper and Four is deepest. Then there's REM when you dream. You pass through these different states in ninety-minute cycles. But any alcohol in the system will stop you moving into stages Three and Four. You won't get that deep sleep that's so important for physical and cognitive repair.'

- Exercise – moderate-to-high-intensity cardio exercise taken early in the day (such as a run, cycle or swim) can have a significant impact on the quality of your sleep that night. 'It will take you less time to get to sleep and you will spend more time in the deeper stages of it.'

- No screens – looking at iPads, PCs or mobile devices in the evening stimulates the brain and doesn't give your body or mind the cues to unwind and relax. 'Reading a printed book offers a much higher degree of positive engagement", says Jackson. 'And it doesn't have the impact of of a lighted screen which will keep your mind in active mode.' Keep phones, screens and any other devices out of the bedroom. 'Even stand-by lights can disturb and interrupt your sleep process, as can digital alarm clocks.' Especially if they're a continual reminder that you're not sleeping – face them away from you or place on the floor.

- Worry list – if you find it difficult to switch off and often fret over a particularly challenging day ahead, list your anxieties. Think about Leahy's productive and unproductive worries while you do this, as outlined in Step 5. 'Keep a notepad and pen by your bed and do this before you settle down to sleep to free up your mind,' suggests Dr Jackson.

4 Listen to what you are hearing and thinking

This step will help you make a connection between what you hear and what you think. We can hear sounds without necessarily engaging with them – notice them but let them pass. Mindfulness helps us view our passing thoughts in a similar way – to recognise them without feeling too absorbed or overwhelmed.

Sounds

1) Sit in a relaxed position in a chair or on the floor and, for a minute or two, bring your focus back to your breath.

2) Bring your attention to any sounds in the room or outside. Be receptive to sounds above and below you, near and far away. Think of pitch, rhythm and loudness. Which sounds are hidden by other sounds? Think about the spaces between each sound.

3) Now notice your natural tendency to label these sounds, how you judge them and how each one can create a story – a woman's shout, a car door slamming.

4) It may be difficult at first but, rather than being tempted to attach a label or explanation to each sound, draw back and refocus. Try to be aware of each sound simply as raw sensation. Focus instead on the ability of being able to hear and on how it's a sense we so often take for granted. After five minutes, let go of your awareness and tune out.

The cycle of sound

I lie on my bed at the top of our house, aware of an endless soundscape outside and in my room. I imagine my hearing is like a long lens, able to zoom in and out of range, catching tiny details miles away and within my own body within the same second. As the thunder of an aeroplane recedes, I note a tinnitus-like ring in my ears, a sharp metal scraping sound from next door's garden, and then my 2-year-old shrieks on the landing below. I become more aware of the space between sounds, the seconds of silence when my hearing comes back to my breathing. Thoughts latch onto different sounds: why so many aeroplanes? I wonder what my daughter looks like, mouth wide open, as she shrieks. Why have I only just noticed an imperceptible ringing in my ears – one to add to my worry audit, at which point the noise becomes more pronounced. So, instead of focusing on this, I try to think about my thoughts chasing sounds and shaping them too, an endless cycle that I've never really been aware of before.

Thoughts

1) Now, for the remaining five minutes, turn your attention to your thoughts. As with the sounds, notice each new one arriving and simply observe them. They may be thoughts from your past – sad, happy, neutral ones; notice them as they come and go.

2) Don't try and control them but let them appear and then pass on their way. Try and see your thoughts as events arising in the mind that stay for a short time and then disperse.

3) Notice when you get caught up with particular thoughts. If you do get drawn in and find it hard to let go of a particular thought, go back to the breath as an anchor to help you re-focus.

Focusing my thoughts is like trying to nail jelly to a wall. But like trying to see those 3D images that were all the rage a while back, the key is relaxing.
Phil, 58

As soon as I try this one out, my mind goes blank too. Thoughts flooded in when I focused on sound, but now I chase after them they're not there. Even my anxious thoughts have gone shy. Is this the point of the exercise, I wonder?

'This is what thoughts are prone to do,' says Professor Williams. 'Proving yet again, it's difficult to control them. Simply notice how they're behaving and observe when they return, which they will do.'

Keep your worries in check
Mindfulness meditations and breathing exercises will help you to engage in the moment and stave off

ruminating about the past and future, but you also need to tackle persistent everyday anxieties, viewing them in a different way to reduce their power. Now it's time to go back and take another look at your worry list with the help of anxiety expert Dr Leahy. He suggests dividing your list into two groups – productive and unproductive worry.

'It's an easy exercise that allows you to see what you do and don't have control over. If you're worrying about a presentation at work the next day, then elements of that are within your control: Are you prepared? Does your PowerPoint cable work? These are details you can do something about. Other questions like "Will my plane crash?" are unproductive, something you have no control over,' explains Dr Leahy.

Productive worry

After you've divided your worries up, can you see a pattern?

This is how Louisa's, 30, looked.

- I worry about work – do colleagues like and respect me? I'd say this is nonproductive. Better to focus on doing my job well rather than trying to second-guess what they think of me.

- My parents – they're healthy now but what about the future as they get older? It makes me anxious to think of them growing more vulnerable. Nonproductive – I should think about spending time with them and enjoying their company now, not continually fretting about a situation that hasn't yet happened.

- I'm 30 years old now but when will I find the time to start a family? Productive – this is becoming more of an issue and could benefit from more discussion with my partner about when would be a good time to think about children.

- Money is the main issue that keeps me awake at night – I constantly worry I won't make it to the end of the month, even though I always do. Productive – I am working through my 5:2 Your Finance steps and taking more control of my money, so I feel less anxious in this area.

- I don't have any health problems but I worry all the time about getting cancer. Nonproductive – apart from staying fit and healthy, there is nothing I can do about this one.

It really helped me to write it all down and get some sort of perspective, to try and focus on what I can do to combat some of my worries and let others go.
Louisa, 30

Dr Leahy also says that this exercise should encourage you to realise your limitations when it comes to unproductive worry. 'People who worry are intolerant of uncertainty. If you can recognise that you have a choice of what you worry about each day, then you can free yourself. I can't worry about when I'm going to die but I can worry about how I live. You can embrace life or embrace worry but it's difficult to do both at the same time.'

Make an appointment with your worries

One day a week, Dr Leahy recommends booking in a set time with your worries. From the moment you wake up, write down your worries and anxieties, big or small. Then let each one go and tell yourself, 'I don't have to engage right now. I'll deal with this at, say, 4 p.m.' By the time you do 'check in', quite a few of them will seem meaningless anyway, says Dr Leahy. Like indigestion, they pass with time. When your scheduled time arrives, sort out your worries into productive and unproductive and what you have left should feel a lot less daunting than when you first started your list in the morning.

6 **Be kind to yourself**

As you move through these steps, you may well feel moments of frustration and negativity; it tends to come with the territory if you're a worrier. A sense of urgency is second nature to most worriers – so much so that we barely notice our tendency to race to the end of any exercise or technique, or our desire for an instant solution, *right now*. When that doesn't happen, frustration and a sense of failure swiftly rush in.

Maybe your mind keeps wandering during the breathing meditation, or so many half-formed worries bubbled up when you tried to do the audit that it was difficult to record them all in a realistic way.

I know that my negative voice will step in as soon as it's able, adept at sabotaging any fresh attempt to break ingrained habits. We blame ourselves, because that's what minds do. 'I can't do this, I may as well give up now. It's not for me.'

'Remember it's not about stopping, resisting or overcoming negative thoughts – although that's a by-product – but actually seeing clearly, looking closely at the mind and how it behaves,' says Professor Williams. 'Being kind to yourself, rather than believing these thoughts, helps you to see them for what they are.'

Reassure yourself, at these points, that this isn't a sign of failure but where you learn most. Acknowledge that it takes hard work to change ingrained habits.

Tuning in to your thoughts

OK, here goes, my first mindfulness meditation. I've set my alarm ten minutes early, before the children are awake, to lie on the floor at the end of my bed. I start concentrating on the toes on my left foot but can't help feeling highly self-conscious. I try to focus on my breath and my first negative thought hijacks me: how farcical this seems. The cynical journalist within can't help mocking what I must look like: a middle-aged woman lying on the floor focusing on her big toe – all I need is wind chimes and a scented candle. It's OK to have these thoughts, I reassure myself, and still benefit from the exercise. Just keep going, I think, and come back to this critical voice later, which I do. Slowly but surely I begin to relax and my inner critic is silenced, for a while.

'This inner critic is the mind trying to bite back', says Professor Williams. 'The "thinking" mind is trying to stay in control. Remember you can't control these thoughts, only understand where they come from and why.'

After my first meditation, it initially felt a bit forced – rather than feel relaxed, I actually felt a wave of anxiety. "I've got so much going on at the moment, this is a pointless indulgence," I couldn't help thinking. But I told myself, "This is a commitment and you have to follow it through." It's a bit like a diet, you're not going to see results straight away but you still have to stick to it. I kept up with the breathing meditations twice a day two times a week and, within a fortnight, I was starting to feel less self-critical, more detached from my thoughts, and that's when I knew something was working.

Pippa, 38

7 Keep worry at bay on the other five days

These exercises are a good way to stay connected to your more intense two-day worry work-outs on your remaining five days, so you can maintain and build on the benefits throughout the week. Best of all, they're short and flexible, able to fit a busy schedule in different environments too. Saying that, don't feel you have to do them every day – the 5:2 Worry Diet is about moderate mindfulness – so fit these in where and when you can.

Three-minute breathing exercise

Minute one

Wherever you're sitting, in a room, on a bus, in a café during a quiet moment, breathe deeply and relax. Close your eyes if you can. Try to block out everything around you and focus only on your thoughts, noticing them as they pass through. Think of clouds, leaves or, as I do, needy children clamouring for your attention. Then simply allow them to move on for now and notice any feelings that arise.

Minute two

Now broaden your focus to include your physical sensations – again simply notice them; allow your mind to drift to different areas of your body and notice the sensations and then allow them to move on.

Minute three

Expand your awareness again to include whatever space you're in. Still try to maintain an awareness of thoughts and physical sensations. Notice what you see and hear; be aware of sensations in that moment. As the third minute ends, bring your attention back to your breath.

> *I tried this during my commute on the train, keeping my earphones on but with no music. It's a good way to zone out the other passengers.*
> Steve, 43

COMMON QUESTIONS

Why do I need to do this?

If you're someone who doesn't suffer from full-blown anxiety but wants to improve their wellbeing and feel more in control of everyday worry.

Which two days should I choose?

Choose two days when you can commit to small windows of time by yourself – Sunday, often a time when worries about the week ahead can begin to mount up, is an ideal day. Follow up with any midweek day.

What should I bear in mind for the other five days?

Be aware of how your two-day practices affect your thoughts for the rest of the week. If there are any persistent anxieties, remind yourself of Dr Robert Leahy's advice to check in with your worries at a particular time – on your chosen Worry Diet days.

I'm finally learning – not always succeeding – to engage less with my worry loop; to let the unproductive anxieties go and make a plan of action for the rest.

Around three weeks in, I begin to imagine my more intrusive thoughts are like tantrum-prone 2-year-olds: the more attention you give them, the more they'll act up. Try not to react and, chances are, they'll pass away. Armed with this analogy, I begin to make real progress, observing my worries without feeling pulled in all directions by them.

> *I've managed to happily co-exist with my inner critic during my meditation exercises, keeping my negative thoughts at arm's length. I find I'm more patient with my partner, appreciating the moment-to-moment pleasure of new activities.*
>
> Pippa, 28

Which other 5:2 life areas combine well with my Worry Diet?

The techniques you'll master during your **Worry** Diet, particularly observing thoughts and impulses without necessarily engaging with them, will be invaluable in many areas: recognising that urge for a glass of wine but then letting the thought go, noticing the desire to check your emails frequently but giving yourself another five minutes to let the moment pass, observing the impulse to click 'Buy' on Amazon or ASOS, or switch on the TV when you don't want to watch anything – but then thinking again. All these make 5:2 Your Worry ideal to combine with 5:2 Your **Drink**, Your **Finance** and Your **Screen** Life.

Slashing your alcohol units, as well as screen-time, will also help aid the deep, restorative sleep that Dr Jackson refers to in Step 3. Match with 5:2 Your **Fitness**, knowing that exercise is proven to reduce the symptoms of stress and anxiety.

FACTS ABOUT WORRYING

- A study from the London School of Economics and Political Science has concluded that some worries, which they describe as 'functional', may be beneficial because it encourages the worrier to find a solution. It cites the fear of being the victim of a crime making you more proactive about your own safety.

- Worriers make better employees and partners, according to research from Carnegie Mellon University in Pennsylvania and the University of North Carolina. People who worry about things that haven't even happened, such as making mistakes at work or being unfaithful, are more conscientious because the anticipation of shame and guilt keeps them in check.

- Intermittent bouts of stress are good for you as they prompt the brain into optimal levels of alertness, behavioural and cognitive performance, as shown in a study at the University of California, Berkeley.

- However, a study jointly run by the University College London and University of Edinburgh shows that those with an anxious disposition are 20 per cent more likely to suffer a heart attack or stroke.

- According to the NHS Information Centre, since the start of the credit crunch in 2008, admissions to hospital with anxiety-related disorders have risen by one third.

● 20.9 per cent of people still rate their anxiety levels at 6 or more out of 10.

● Mental illnesses, such as depression and anxiety, cost the UK economy some £80 million annually. On average we spend two hours of our day worrying, which adds up to a worrying five years of our lives.

● Stress and anxiety have a major impact on your ability to work. A major study of tens of thousands of individual GPs' sick notes found that 35 per cent of those surveyed were given for 'mild to moderate mental health disorders', such as depression, anxiety and stress.

5:2

YOUR ENVIRONMENT

LIFE BEFORE MY 5:2 ENVIRONMENT FIX

When I first began to reflect on changes I could make to my life twice a week to help the environment, I must admit to feeling daunted. 'I'm saving the planet on Mondays and Fridays' could sound suspiciously trite. The danger can be that with such a vast subject, the more you find out the more you can feel powerless to make a difference.

Whereas the 5:2 approach to other areas, such as diet, fitness or alcohol, has measurable results that you can see week by week, helping the environment creates a much broader challenge. It almost certainly requires a new set of habits if, like I was, you're still buying green beans from Kenya and blueberries from Poland out of season and forgetting, yet again, to take your plastic bags to the supermarket. And, beyond that, it demands a shift in mindset, believing that leadership can start from one individual action; that if enough people behave in a certain way, bigger changes are possible.

I always struggled with the idea that environmental decisions can be about making a stand, rather than an actual change. Take flying: when I decided to take the train to France last year, I looked up the emissions saved by not travelling by plane: 250kg/CO_2. By going on Eurostar I was, satisfyingly, reducing the CO_2 output of the journey by 85 per cent. Except that I wasn't because, in reality, the plane still took off, still created the same emissions. My behaviour would only have been effective if enough people had made the same choice as me.

> *I decided to stop flying because I wanted to take a personal action. As an individual you can feel very helpless, but by doing this I feel I'm taking control. It takes the pressure of the enormity of what's happening if you can think, "At least I'm doing this" – and you don't know where change starts. It could lead to something; it could be a springboard that eventually appeals to someone. You can't rule out that possibility – but you can if you do nothing.*
> Beth, 60

To feel committed, I realise that I need to view my individual actions twice a week as part of a bigger picture: committing to a 5:2 approach to your environment may not feel like a substantial contribution initially, but if enough people take even this moderate action, the impact will be significant. As the philosopher Edmund Burke wrote, 'Nobody made a greater mistake than he who did nothing because he could do only a little.'

Similarly, I'm conscientious about recycling, but whenever I try to imagine what really happens to all those empty cartons and loo rolls, who sorts them out and where they go, I draw a blank: I can't quantify how much, if at all, this will help the environment. If I knew how it *really* worked I'm sure I'd be committed at a deeper level. On my first 5:2 Environment Fix day, I find myself phoning my local council, who point me to a detailed explanation on their website of each recycling stage, where it happens and the environmental benefits of this service: at least I feel much more aware of how my contribution is part of a larger and important process.

This isn't just about increased awareness of environmental matters, although that's crucial too, but thinking in a different way, being less passive and more curious, keener to take control. As Mike Berners-Lee, author of *How Bad Are Bananas?*, says, 'If you get into the habit of thinking about what lies behind a lot of what you consume, you do go through a gate in your head and find different things appealing.' If you begin to find out more, what you discover will have a knock-on effect way beyond the confines of two days each week.

My assumption, pre-5:2, was that making tiny changes would feel like a false investment, like turning off lights and having showers instead of baths. Is it worth sweating the small stuff, I'd wonder? After research and talking to experts, I now know the answer is, yes – even more so if you can measure it: see Step 2 on charting your progress. There are other unexpected benefits too: the satisfaction of feeling more aware and knowledgeable, as well increasing your wellbeing. See Step 7: make it a joy, not a duty.

Before you embark on your two-day environmental diet, you need to know what's worth giving up and what isn't. Read about and research environmental initiatives in your area. Also a good place to start is Berners-Lee's book, where he calculates the real impact of everything we do and buy and advises you on where to 'pick your battles'. There are also useful websites that can help

you find out more about your carbon footprint – www.footprint.
wwf.org.uk is a constructive one.

Make sure the changes you make are worthwhile as well as
satisfying. As Berners-Lee says, 'It's very demoralising to go to a
lot of effort to give something up thinking it makes a difference
but then discover that it doesn't.'

I somehow felt that behaving differently would involve personal
sacrifice and a modicum of pain. But this sort of attitude, as I was
about to discover, is doomed to failure. Think about it from a new
perspective, says Berners-Lee. 'Caring about climate change and
green living gets framed in all the wrong ways. Your goal should
be no hit to wellbeing, and if your wellbeing has gone down then
you're not doing it right.' I'll raise a glass of organic wine to that.

MAKING THE 5:2 CONNECTION

Initially I worried that the environment was too vast an area to
work neatly in the 5:2 ratio. So I was pleasantly surprised when
I started talking to environmental experts and campaigners who
were extremely enthusiastic about implementing changes twice
a week.

Berners-Lee was keen about the impact on diet. 'If you only
go veggie for two days each week, your life would become more
interesting.'

'If you were to apply yourself twice a week, you'll build up
overall awareness,' says Joanna Yarrow, green lifestyle specialist,
and author of *How to Reduce Your Carbon Footprint: 365 Practical
Ways to Make a Real Difference.*

Julia Hailes, campaigning consultant and author of *The New
Green Consumer Guide*, agrees, 'It's about breaking habits two
days a week and finding you can manage perfectly well without
certain things; less heating or, say, never using paper napkins, and

realising it's perfectly comfortable, that you're happy to make it a permanent change.'

Which is why the 5:2 Environment Fix is ideal for those who are looking to make small yet realistic changes that can bring other bonuses into play.

THE 5:2 ENVIRONMENT FIX; aims and benefits

- A simple – and measurable – way to reduce your carbon footprint by changing habits twice a week.

- It will demand you look at your life in a new way; that you become more thoughtful and responsible, questioning and challenging, not just environmentally but more generally too.

- Helping the environment is one benefit of focusing on this 5:2 life area, but there will be a more holistic payoff too: you'll feel fitter (driving less), healthier (eating less meat), wealthier (spending less) and happier (you're bound to when you combine these three!).

- Gain more satisfaction knowing you're focusing on the issues that can really make a difference.

- These changes won't feel like a sacrifice or a compromise – they'll improve your daily life, not diminish it.

- You'll appreciate the contrasts in your lifestyle, become more aware of how one way of living makes the other more enjoyable.

- You can still enjoy and savour those habits you sacrifice twice a week – driving, eating meat, spending money, even flying – if it's a much rarer event.

GETTING STARTED ON THE 5:2 ENVIRONMENT FIX

The following steps will help you to reflect on your attitudes and values, and how committed you are to environmental issues, and allow you to establish some goals that you can measure. Your two-day fix will be geared to areas that can really make an impact, honing in on achievable tasks. Key to this approach is the emphasis on only making changes that will enhance wellbeing, make life more interesting and create benefits in all of your other 5:2 life areas.

SEVEN STEPS TO MAKE THE 5:2 ENVIRONMENT FIX WORK FOR YOU

1 Do a green audit

Be clear about your motivations and what you'd really like to get out of your 5:2 Environment Fix. As a starting point, look at what you're doing already:

- Do you drive more than you walk?

- Are you aware of conserving energy at home?

- Do you read about environmental issues in the newspapers, magazines, online?

- How much do you recycle?

- Do you shop ethically or think about the history of what you're buying; do you consider how much workers were paid to make that pair of jeans, or how far that punnet of strawberries has flown?

- Are you part of an environmental group, joining something that helps the community?

Is it enough? What would you like to do more? Sit down with a pen and paper and make a list of environmental improvements you feel would be realistic, and that feel important to you right now.

State your reasons and don't worry how small-scale they may sound.

I would love to be more green, be more aware of what impact my lifestyle has on the environment. I have recently got a car for the school run and feel so guilty – I want to aim to use it only when absolutely necessary, like when it's pouring down, not just when I can't be bothered to walk. My motivation is fear – all the talk of carbon fuels running out in my lifetime scares me silly, not just for me but for my daughters. I fear that the green alternatives just won't be able to keep up with demands and wonder what will happen then?

Fran, 38

My own tiny goal is to rid myself of my plastic bag cupboard. Currently I have one so rammed with them that they tumble out whenever I open the door. I am aiming to whittle them down to just a few by taking them out with me – not just when I do the supermarket shop. I always seem to accumulate them because I haven't got one on me so now I'm keeping a store in the car too. When I've got rid of them I'll use my sturdier bags (that are currently holding a million bags in them). My motivation is seeing the "witches' knickers" of old plastic bags caught in the branches of trees near where I live – so awful.

Janice, 53

As part of my list of improvements, I decide that my commitment for the first two weeks of my 5:2 Environment Fix will be reading and researching online, increasing my environmental awareness twice a week. I'm convinced that this is key to then making worthwhile practical changes and feeling confident about my choices.

Now you have a better understanding of your motivations and what you would like to achieve, you need to be clear about what parts of your lifestyle are non-negotiable and what aspects you would be willing to change and try something different.

These are some of the areas you could think about and consider the alternatives:

- Driving to work

- Flying abroad for work and holiday

- Shopping at supermarkets

- Regularly updating your wardrobe

- Eating meat more than three days a week

- Buying fruit and vegetables out of season

- Throwing away food you don't eat

- Buying on impulse, rather than buying to last

- Drinking bottled water

Ideally, discuss your responses to these comments with a friend or partner.

My partner drives a long distance to work and is resistant to any alternatives such as car-sharing, because he needs to drive to appointments during his day, but he is open to working from home when possible. He also is very keen on meat and finds a meal without it a hardship, whereas I used to be vegetarian for seventeen years and would happily go back to it. So there is some friction in our approach to being green – depending on how much it impinges on our lifestyles, it seems. But two days a week doesn't seem too challenging, especially if I use my Madhur Jaffrey World Vegetarian cookbook.'

Kevin, 54

2 Habits you can measure

On a 5:2 diet, your simple goal is to lose weight and you can measure it easily by stepping on the scales. For each pound that falls, you feel closer to your goal. Being more mindful about your environment twice a week could be less tangible but, says Yarrow, it really doesn't have to be. 'Measuring your progress is still very possible,' she says. 'As long as you choose areas that are quantifiable.' In other words, know which battles are worth fighting and track your progress.

Energy

You can cut back on your energy usage twice a week in the same way that you reduce your calories. Rather than weighing scales, you'll need a wireless home energy monitoring product like the 'owl' – see www.theowl.com. This is a compact device that will tell you how much electricity you're using each hour, from your toaster to your tumble drier. 'If you're boiling your kettle, it will tell you the cost and may make you think twice about perhaps having a glass of tap water instead,' says Yarrow. 'Men in particular get obsessed with these devices once they can see what a difference each appliance makes – children enjoy them as well.'

When I get my 'owl' through the post, I try to turn everything off in the house to stop the counter ticking up endlessly. It is tricky, and it makes me aware of how much I have on standby – such as the dishwasher that's flashing and beeping to let me know it's finished and the phone charger that is still plugged into the socket and is warm to the touch. I feel like the energy police, snooping around trying to find something plugged in.

On your first 5:2 Environment Fix day, make a note of how much electricity you use. On every other 5:2 day that follows, see how much you can cut down. Looking at this twice weekly, you'll build up an awareness that will affect the way you think about energy use for the rest of the week too.

'Twice a week, choose three pieces of electrical equipment you can rely on and turn off the rest,' suggests Julia Hailes. 'It may not be totally easy but it is realistic.' And it's a great challenge that will make you appreciate your electrical products for the rest of the week too. 'Make sure your equipment is not on standby and everything is switched off.' Use your energy monitor to surprise you with the saving,' she adds.

For the more resilient, try turning off your heat once a week as a challenge, regardless of the weather outside.

The upside of cutting down on electricity just twice a week is that if you were using a meter and cutting down every day, you would probably stop noticing it. This way, you can ask yourself how much better or worse your monitor is looking and feel the contrast between your energy 'off' and 'on' days. Either way it's a win: for example, you can appreciate and r elish a warmer house on the other five days after two days of denial, or discover that it's no sacrifice at all and use less electricity and gas all week round.

Drying my hair was something I did without thinking at least four times a week, but using the smart meter and seeing the counter move so quickly while the hairdryer was on was an eye-opener. I didn't realise that it uses more energy than a tumble drier – which I don't have for environmental reasons, ironically! I can easily let my hair dry naturally after I've been to the gym after work.

Philippa, 27

Travel

You can cut your fuel use by 30 per cent, according to Yarrow, if you follow these simple and measurable steps twice a week:

- Check your car for ways of reducing 'drag', which creates resistance, uses more fuel and therefore increases fuel costs: does it have a roof rack or storage box that could be removed and stored?

- Make sure your car tyres are pumped up – driving on softer ones works the engine harder.

- Use air-conditioning as little as possible – another drain on fuel.

- Watch your speed. 'Faster driving uses more fuel,' says Yarrow. 'Keeping to fifty miles per hour uses 30 per cent less fuel than seventy miles per hour.'

- If there's a route you do regularly, see how much fuel you use and test yourself on a 5:2 driving day after you've combined some of these tips. Keep a tally of how much you use before and after you start for the first week or two, and then check regularly to see if there's a difference.

I'm a classic middle-lane hogger on the motorway – driving at seventy to eighty miles per hour, but I tried switching to the slow lane for two days a week and it didn't actually take that much longer since there were traffic jams anyway. I got that tortoise-and-the-hare superior feeling when I caught up with the speed-freaks.
　　Justin, 47

- Service your car regularly – an inefficient engine can reduce your car's fuel efficiency by at least 10 per cent.

- On one or both of your 5:2 days, think about alternative travel options – car-sharing, public transport, walking or cycling. 'Replace a five-mile car trip with a bike ride once a week and you'll prevent around a hundred kilograms of CO_2 emissions a year', says Yarrow.

- Keep track of your petrol receipts: how much fuel have you used, per week, over the last two or three months? Keep a weekly record after you start your 5:2 Environment Fix and make a note of 'before' and 'after' as an incentive.

I have a small car (a VW Polo) and use it for the school run – a trip of around a mile. I fill up once a month at a cost of £40. I tried walking with the children for two days a week and this month the petrol gauge is still a quarter full, saving me £10. The children were annoyed at first – it's not even 'Walk to School Week' – but they have come round to it and ironically we don't have to leave so early in the mornings to get a place in the school car park.
　　Theresa, 43

If possible, let your children cycle or walk to school – according to recent research carried out by two Danish universities, children who are driven to school by car, or who travel by public transport, don't perform as well in tests measuring their concentration levels as those who do a bit of exercise on their way in.

3 Think about how you eat

A week or two before you start your Environment Fix, get into the habit of tallying your receipts and keep a 'consumption' diary of what you spend and where – which shops do you tend to go to most? Local markets, supermarkets or shopping online? You could use your money diary from Step 1 of 5:2 Your Finance. Make a note of which types of foods are most likely to get thrown out at the end of week, or end up festering at the back of the fridge. When you begin your Environment Fix, carry on with your diary, and after a week or two compare and contrast your entries with your food shopping patterns before you started your Environment Fix. Hopefully there should be a satisfying contrast, even over just two days each week.

Similarly, before you change your shopping behaviour, make a note of how many bags of rubbish you throw out each day or each week so that you can keep tabs on your progress once you start.

My consumption diary was helpful in that it really made me aware of the things that I'd prefer not to dwell on, such as not being bothered to recycle the envelopes with plastic windows in them and the amount of food we waste. The vegetable drawers in our fridge are a dark cave of doom. Normally I cram in the fresh stuff on top and daren't venture below,

but I made myself excavate it so I could start from scratch, knowing what I had. No need to buy any more celery – I buy a whole head but only need one or two sticks to make stock and the rest goes off. I've now made a vat of stock and frozen it. Knowing I was actively trying to avoid throwing things away became a challenge – how can I use that one remaining beetroot? Beetroot and feta salad, that's how.
Imogen, 55

Once you've started the fix, you should be aiming for a 10 per cent reduction in how much you consume and in the cost of your food bills, if you're following the steps ahead conscientiously.

How and what we eat even twice a week can make a significant impact on our carbon footprint. This means that, at least three times each day (unless you're on a 5:2 diet), we all have the opportunity to make an impact. Between 20 to 30 per cent of most people's carbon footprint is created by their food choices – that figure is higher depending on how much food you throw away.

According to a report by the United Nations in September 2013, each year around a third of all food – that's about 1.3 billion tonnes – is wasted, along with all the energy, water and chemicals needed to produce and then dispose of it. They have estimated that the carbon footprint of wasted food is equivalent to 3.3 billion tons of carbon dioxide per year, and have recommended that consumers in the developed world eat smaller portions and make better use of leftovers. 'If we stopped wasting food, throwing away what we don't eat, the climate saving in the UK would be the equivalent of taking one in five cars off the road,' says Yarrow.

According to recent figures from Tesco, in the first six months of 2013 its stores and distribution centres generated 28,500 tonnes of food waste. It also estimated that across the UK food industry, 68% of salad to be sold in bags is currently wasted – 35% of it thrown out by customers.

Why does throwing food away create CO_2?

When you throw food in your bin it's transported to landfill. Anything organic that decomposes with little to no oxygen creates methane – one of the strongest climate gases and around twenty-one times more potent than carbon dioxide. Something as benign as an apple core can be a climate threat, if it's allowed to rot anaerobically i.e. with low to no oxygen. If it's composted with access to oxygen, it can break down without creating methane.

Remember, wasting less food in the first place will make a more significant change than how you dispose of it. Berners-Lee says that composting is preferable to landfill but it still won't allow you to escape from the fact that the carbon footprint has already been set in motion by producing the food in the first place.

Food

On both your 5:2 environment days, think creatively and set in motion these small changes:

- Cook in batches twice a week to last you for at least another two or three meals, using up leftover ingredients in the fridge and less electricity. 'Rather than thinking of this as a sacrifice on your 5:2 environment day, as in "Oh, this is lentil day", think of it as twice a week when you can try a new recipe, and make one of those evenings a time when you have friends around to try it out', suggests Yarrow.

- Don't waste what you buy: eat everything on your plate and save leftovers. 'Eradicating waste is worth a 25 per cent saving for the average shopper,' says Berners-Lee.

- Go online and search for batch recipe ideas by ingredient – try Abel and Cole (www.abelandcole.co.uk) who have recipes listed by vegetable; there are over thirty delicious ones for the humble broccoli alone. And their weekly veg boxes come with handy recipe ideas too.

Batch winner

Usually, I leave most of the cooking to my husband but now I'm starting my 5:2 Environment Fix, I decide to test out batch cooking – there's something satisfying about cooking in volume. For lazy chefs, like me, it means less effort overall, always knowing that there's something ready and waiting. You'll spend and waste less too – the ultimate 5:2 win.

Every Saturday I have a vegetable box delivered, so Sunday evening is all about batch-cooking the contents to make sure everything is used up, which means I've got most meals sorted for the rest of the week.

There's something very satisfying about having a big bowl in the fridge that you can dip into and eat hot or cold.

It's great fun getting creative with the veg you're sent – last week I got adventurous with roasted butternut squash and chard! In just one and a half hours I can make enough soup (I raid the fridge for ALL leftovers from the past week, as anything tastes good when liquidised with chicken stock), bean/couscous/quinoa salads, coleslaw, and Bolognese sauce to last till Friday. I even pack my husband off to work with a thermos of soup and a salad to make sure nothing's wasted.

By the end of the week, anything not used up (bar the salads), is frozen.

This means I only really cook properly on Sundays and Thursdays, as usually we're out on Fridays and Saturdays, so for Monday to Wednesday, all our lunches and dinners are pre-made; which, including lunches, can be more than ten meals. It never gets boring either, because each vegetable box is different, so if you get imaginative and mix-and-match your recipes, you often come up with some amazing meals.

That's a massive saving in time, effort, money and energy used. I also usually make Mondays and Wednesdays my 'fast' days, so I'm eating less anyway, and anything not used on those days gets eaten on Friday or Saturday if we don't go out.

There's something enormously satisfying about batch-cooking, not least because it's good fun, environmentally friendly and frees you up to do other things besides standing over a stove. And for someone who doesn't especially like cooking or is even any good at it, that's reason enough.

- Get together with a neighbour or friend and buy in bulk or from a local food co-operative – for more details look online: www. sustainweb.org/foodcoops/ is a good place to start. Keep an eye out for local farmers' markets and food festivals that might offer some good deals on bulk buys at the end of the day.

- You may not have space, or time, to grow your own vegetables, but a herb box on your window sill is a decent compromise, saving on processing, packaging and transport.

I made a pact with myself to plant herbs on my first 5:2 week. That was six weeks ago, and I use them all the time. I've now spotted a tiny patch in our garden where I'm going to grow potatoes. I've been reading all about how to do it. There are environmental benefits but, just as importantly, I've created another hobby and interest.
   Rose, 61

- Make your own compost – find out more about how to build your own compost bin on www.recyclenow.com, or kits are readily available online or from the recycling department of many local councils.

Be a 5:2 seasonarian

If you're trying to keep it simple, eating what's in season and buying locally grown can be very effective. Take, for example, local asparagus, which creates 125 grams of CO_2e^* in terms of production and transport, compared to the same pack flown from Peru in January which, says Berners-Lee, accounts for 3.5 kilograms of CO_2e.

---

* CO_2e, where 'e' is equivalent, is Mike Berners-Lee's measure: it means the total climate-change impact of all greenhouse gases.

Still, it's not always as simple as switching closer to home – local produce can sometimes have the same carbon footprint as food shipped in from thousands of miles away because of the pressure on farmers to grow crops out of season in heated greenhouses, using more energy than growing them in hotter climates and flying them over. However, if you focus on what's in season, you'll be cutting your footprint by as much as 600–700 kilograms a year.

Consider ordering a seasonal organic vegetable box that delivers within a local radius, and enjoy the challenge of cooking a variety of different offerings each week. Keep an eye on what to look out for seasonally at local markets and in your supermarket by checking websites such as www.eatseasonably. co.uk/ what-to-eat-now/calendar/ and www.whats-in-season. com.

The urge to buy unseasonal fruit seems especially strong for me at special occasions – Valentine's Day means strawberries, dinner parties need grapes for the cheese board – but I'm trying to find alternatives such as rhubarb fool and radishes.

Drink

Liquid is heavy, whether it's beer, wine or spirits, so think about how far it's travelled before it reaches your glass – what's important is road miles within your country and where it's produced. Locally produced wine, beer or even spirits (I'm lucky enough to have an independent distillery at the end of my street – no road miles to worry about for my local bottle of gin) can cut the footprint by a quarter.

Track down your local microbrewery. To find one near you, a good place to start is www.camra.org.uk/locale.

I made cider from our windfall apples and it was amazingly drinkable. Freezing the apples first makes it a lot easier to get the juice from them. It works out at just a few pence per pint too.

Steve, 44

I find it tough not buying our weekly stock of six 1-litre bottles of fizzy water. I know I've been seduced by the Italian design more than anything – it still amounts to a lot of plastic, processing and polythene. I stick to tap water instead and save around £65 a month. Or you could buy a water carbonator such as a Sodastream. They start at around £50, but the cannisters cost less than £10 to refill and make about 60 litres of carbonated water – working out around 16p per litre.

4. Be a 5:2 Veggie

There's no escaping the fact that eating meat contributes significantly to your carbon footprint, by around 10 per cent, according to Berners-Lee. Global meat production has proliferated in the last fifty years, meaning that the average British carnivore eats around 11,000 animals in their lifetime, each making huge demands on land, fuel and water supplies. There's also the unsavoury downside of all those greenhouse gases produced by livestock – in other words, cow farts – contributing to around 37 per cent of methane emissions. Cattle production contributes to around 18 per cent of greenhouse gases worldwide, more than road transport.

'By avoiding meat altogether', says Yarrow, 'you can cut the CO_2 associated with your diet by about half.' So by giving it a miss twice a week, you can slash your CO_2 food contribution by almost a quarter.

Seven days a week may feel too extreme, but two days a week to change your diet is realistic. Why not make sure one of your 5:2 veggie days is on Monday and tie in with the Meat Free Monday campaign (www.meatfreemondays.com), which believes that 'One day a week can make a world of difference.' In which case, think what two could do.

This trend of eating meat on a less regular and more flexible basis has been gathering momentum for a while now, thanks partly to carnivore chefs like Hugh Fearnley-Whittingstall who can see the health and environmental advantages, as can Simon Hopkinson who says, 'It's not a militant or radical approach, it's just about not always necessarily having meat,' which sums up the 5:2 veggie ratio perfectly.

Eating more vegetables than meat means not having to make drastic changes to your – or your children's – eating habits, or feeling you're on an extreme crusade. It's a moderate shift that is clearly successful already – the Vegetarian Research Group found that 23 million people follow a 'vegetarian-inclined diet', compared to 7.3 million full-time veggies.

'Two days is enough to introduce yourself to a different way of eating. You may find yourself rethinking your diet,' says Yarrow. 'It tunes you in to the fact that a diet without meat can be satisfying. On other days, think of meat as a garnish – bacon on your salad – rather than always the main course.'

> *I can't abide those vegetarian equivalents such as veggie sausages and mince, so I make meals that don't have meat in normally, such as margarita pizza and spinach-and-ricotta cannelloni.*
> Joanna, 29

' *I do love meat but I also worry about the environmental impact of beef and the amount of animal fat I eat. So twice a week I've been building up a repertoire of vegetarian meals. I think I'd find it too difficult all week to find different recipes that I felt confident about but for two days it's fun, easy and it keeps you interested.* '

Kirsty, 40

5. Buy less, spend less, buy better

Everything that you buy has taken energy to produce, process, package and transport. Another top priority for your 5:2 Environment Fix days is to reflect more deeply on where an item may have been produced, in what conditions, and how far it may have travelled. As Berners-Lee says, 'Think a bit more, follow the trail in your mind and wonder what lies behind whatever you want to buy – there's a whole history that may not be good, and you're buying into it if you decide to make a purchase. If you don't, you're taking yourself out of the market, which will make an impact.'

For this reason, I no longer go to certain clothes shops, even though my daughter nags me that we can buy much more for our money there. I explain the reasoning and I offer to buy her one item for the cost of about three elsewhere, knowing it has been produced in better conditions, is much better quality and will last longer too.

Remember that recycling isn't enough, although it can make an impact on the waste you create, but it's one end of a consumer chain that begins with production. We're still producing and buying more year-on-year and that's one reason we have to recycle. Starting at the source and consuming less in the first place is a more carbon-friendly approach. Check out www.recyclenow.com to find the more unusual items that can be recycled.

Think about your purchasing decisions on your 5:2 days, advises Yarrow. 'Make sure your weekly shop has recycled products in it in the first place – loo paper and kitchen roll – and look for less packaging.'

Combine your 5:2 'buy less' days with your restricted-spending days on the 5:2 Money Diet: leave the house with less money and no credit cards. When you really want to buy something, ask yourself why, and find useful psychological strategies to step away from that purchase in 5:2 Your Finance.

Focus on buying more rarely but better quality and you'll waste less. 'I had a choice with my sofa recently, whether to re-cover it or buy another. We refurbished it for much less than the cost of a new one but, as importantly, it was a satisfying thing to do. You end up with a more interesting home, and wardrobe,' says Berners-Lee.

> I waited for eight years to replace my laptop and I've bought myself one that is top-of-the range and I don't have a problem with that. I want the best quality I can find because I know I'll hang on to it for years. Like the last one, I'll get it mended and upgraded a few times. Hopefully it will be with me for a long time and I'll also get that extra satisfaction knowing I'm really annoying computer companies by hanging on to one model – it's not what they want at all which is the big win for me!
>
> Ben, 42

> Instead of buying ready-made curtains from the high street, I bought fabric from our little independent fabric

*shop and made them myself. It wasn't rocket science – very
straightforward in fact, and it felt good to be supporting our
local businesses.*

Marie, 37

Spend money on experiences rather than 'things', as long
as they don't involve air flight! A survey four years ago at San
Francisco State University showed that life experiences, rather
than possessions, lead to greater happiness. According to Ryan
Howell, assistant professor of psychology, the study 'demonstrates
that experiential purchases, such as a meal out or theatre tickets,
result in increased wellbeing because they satisfy higher-order
needs, specifically the need for social connectedness and
vitality – a feeling of being alive.'

In a paper out in 2013, 'When Wanting Is Better Than Having',
Professor Marsha Richins from the University of Missouri, wrote:
'Although materialists still experience positive emotions after
making a purchase, they are less intense than before they actually
acquire a product.' In three separate studies, 'materialists' report
significantly more happiness thinking about their purchase
beforehand than after they bought it.

6 Reject fast fashion

We throw away around 1.5 million tonnes of clothing
each year. According to Oxfam, 9,513 garments
were thrown into landfill every five minutes, adding up to one
billion items per year – the equivalent of one in four garments
sold. Meanwhile manmade fibres will live on for centuries.

Think about alternatives to fast fashion and buy clothes that
are durable. 'On one of your 5:2 environment days, organise a

clothes swap with friends,' suggests Yarrow. 'Or have an evening together where you "upcycle" clothes to create something new.' For more ideas, visit www.upcyclethat.com

Devise a different wardrobe-related activity for each of your 5:2 days. It could be just washing your clothes at a low temperature and not using the tumble dryer. For the satisfaction of knowing what it's saved you, check your energy monitor.

I found that buying small accessories can make discarded clothes completely wearable again. Extra thick black tights mean my tailored tweed mini-skirt has a bit more life in it, and looks good with boots. A leopard-skin belt has also updated an old black dress I had in the back of my wardrobe.

Look on one of your two days as an opportunity to develop a new hobby – sewing, knitting or crafting. Danielle Proud's *House Proud: Hip Craft for the Modern Homemaker* is a great introduction.

Scour vintage and charity shops for a bargain – give yourself a price limit and see what you can afford. For the best charity shops out there, explore the best residential areas where you get a better class of reject. You can also perk up tired, washed-out clothes with a dye. On one of my 5:2 environment days, I dig out a pair of old grey jeans and they're transformed into jet black skinnies with one wash cycle and a £5 dye. On a Saturday morning, we collect half-a-dozen old t-shirts and vests together and tie-dye them in bright colours – the children loved picking out different dyes and now wear their transformed tops as nightclothes. It's fun experimenting with different tie-dye patterns.

Check for low-CO_2 textiles such as fleeces recycled from plastic bottles and organic cotton (nonorganic cotton is the world's most polluting crop, requiring 50,000 tonnes of pesticides each year), hemp fibre or bamboo – a hectare of bamboo absorbs up to 2 tonnes of CO_2 every year, says Yarrow.

Recycle your unwanted clothes that can't be swapped, sent to charity or 'upcycled'. Look into local schemes – your council is often a good place to start. www.rag-bag.co.uk organise collections of clothes through schools and clubs and pay them for every kilogram recycled.

7. Make it a joy not a duty

Look for changes that will make a difference in terms of reducing your carbon footprint but will also make life more interesting in some way, not difficult and onerous. If you re-educate your mind, you can find that behaving in a different way doesn't feel like an enormous effort. Call it selfish altruism if you like: you'll be helping the planet, but in a way that creates personal benefits too. Even just twice a week, you need a sense of novelty, challenge and satisfaction to make the habit stick.

In Berners-Lee's case, where these goals intersect is travel. He knew he could reduce his carbon footprint by cycling to his local train station and taking his fold-up bike to work. 'I enjoy it so much that I sometimes make a point of taking a longer route to work on my bike. I also save money and it keeps me fit – I do the odd fell-running race and I'm much better at it as a result of cycling, and running for the train. My life is so much better because I took that one decision to drive less. Sometimes I do take my car and I lift-share on the days I fancy a chat. There are much better ways of doing things but they all require a bit of habit changing. But this has been an easy one to form because it wasn't a nasty medicine, and that's the key.'

Aim for 'synergistic goals'

Synergy, where the sum is greater than its parts or, in simple terms, 2 + 2 = 5, is one of those much overused business terms, but it is useful in this context. Making positive steps to consume less and conserve more, and simply being more curious about how your everyday actions affect the environment, will help to create a cascade of mutually beneficial goals across your 5:2 life areas.

So, if your one simple goal is to walk or cycle everywhere two days a week, you'll be gaining green points, as well as scoring highly in fitness, worry, finance, productivity, and relationships (read about the benefits of walking in 5:2 Your Relationship, and its impact on creativity as well). All of these will disproportionately boost wellbeing, too. The 5:2 linked benefits rectangle below shows how achieving one step creates another benefit.

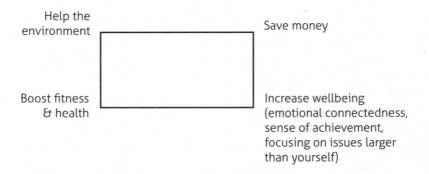

The ultimate 5:2 goal is to think of – and to put into practice – actions that match all four points. For example:

- Walking to work, or part of the way, and/or walking your children to school

- Cycling

- Eating less meat

- Gardening, composting, planting vegetables

> *Growing veg in my garden has been the best thing I've done in years. It's so therapeutic pottering around after a day at work; it keeps me fit and you can't get much more locally sourced than your back garden.*
>
> Mary, 59

Take pleasure from 'beating the system'

One immense satisfaction that you can derive from being more environmentally aware, as well as helping the planet, of course, is that smug sense of somehow outwitting the 'system'; paying less to the multinationals, be they supermarkets or energy companies; 'winning' through ingenuity and guile.

> *In the summer, I turned off the boiler and had enough hot water for four or five days. It's good for saving energy but I can't kid myself that's the reason I felt so satisfied. It was more to do with that feeling of not being fleeced, of opting out and being a bit more self-sufficient. It made me feel very clever, which is a nice feeling. I'll definitely be doing it again.*
>
> Betty, 63

> *I'm quite shy but I persuaded myself to approach someone from my village who goes to the same gym as me. We now go together in one car – and as a bonus have started going to different exercise classes so it's been a good social experiment too.*
>
> Abi, 35

Be nice to yourself

As your 5:2 Environment Fix days turn into weeks, reward yourself, recommends Yarrow. 'Think about a buddy system, just like people do with the 5:2 diet. Get a friend on board and then have some sort of party or celebration at the end of six months when you've stuck to it. Show off your new figure thanks to all that walking and cycling and, with what you've saved on the electricity bill, splash out on some lovely local booze.'

> *Once the novelty had worn off, it felt a little harder sticking to my new green ways – especially when the weather turned colder and I was still walking to the train station – but I was determined to continue as I told myself that even the small changes make a difference.*
> Tess, 38

Enjoy life more by not flying

In Berners-Lee's book, *How Bad Are Bananas?*, he advises readers to find the area where you can quantify maximum return for your efforts. Top of his and every environmentalist's list is one simple maxim: fly as little as you can.

Of course, this isn't something you'll be planning specifically during your twice-weekly Environment Fix, but it's one issue you can reflect on over your two days; try and think about alternative options for work and holiday travel.

If you're in any doubt, air travel accounts for around 10 per cent of manmade climate emissions and that's increasing by 5 per cent a year. As Berners-Lee points out in his book, the average long-haul flight from Hong Kong to London burns through 116 tons of fuel over its 9,700-kilometre journey. As the fuel burns, he says, it creates three times its weight in CO_2 – and because it happens at high altitude, the impact is much greater.

Think of the upsides of travelling by train rather than flying, including saving money and time wasted at airports. Check out www.seat61.com for some very inspiring figures on the amount of emissions you save by taking the train rather than flying. For example, flying from London to Nice will incur 250kg/CO_2 compared to 36kg/CO_2 by taking the train: an 85 per cent saving.

> *One recent summer holiday we took the children on a train ride, walked and camped. It was a simple low-key holiday that the children still talk about more than any other. We didn't have to waste a day travelling, waiting around, getting organised. We just walked out of the back door, jumped on train and didn't plan ahead. If you fly, in contrast, you're a slave while you're in transit, a prisoner at airports wasting all that precious holiday time. Nothing can beat our local holiday. When I do fly, I make sure it's a special occasion and that I spend longer there.*
>
> Mike, 35

> *My husband and I never fly and that's an environmental decision – we feel strongly it's the worst thing you can do. But it's easy to commit to because the alternative is far more enjoyable. We regularly take the train across Europe for breaks and summer holidays now. In practice there are mixed advantages – travelling from Budapest to Warsaw recently was tiring, probably more so than flying. But the benefits far outweighed this – the thought of the actual journey was very exciting, very much part of the holiday rather than a means to an end. We got to know far more about that part of Western Europe, how immense it was, and the people who lived there – it was a much more immersive experience rather than that awful constrained feeling of being on a plane.*
>
> Jan, 58

COMMON QUESTIONS

Which two days should I choose to focus on the environment?

Make sure one of your environment days is on Mondays and gain instant membership to Meat Free Monday if you become a 5:2 vegetarian.

What other 5:2 life areas can I combine with the Environment Fix?

5:2 Your **Money**: you'll be saving money by consuming less and you may also want to consider looking into ethical investments. If you manage to save enough and fancy a few stocks and shares thanks to your 5:2 Money Diet days, then think about Aberdeen, F&C and Jupiter who all have funds that apply ethical or environmental criteria, and the ethical building society, Ecology Building Society (www.ecology.co.uk). Cycling and walking as part of your seven environment steps make 5:2 Your **Environment** a good companion to 5:2 Your **Fitness**, and walking more to cut down on your carbon footprint connects beneficially with 5:2 Your **Relationship** – a key activity than can boost communication and shared intimacy. It also complements 5:2 Your **Worry**. If you fret about the bigger issues like global warming, this may help you feel more proactive about taking control. It may also be interesting to reflect on to what extent environment is a productive or nonproductive worry, as per the exercise on p.226 of 5:2 Your Worry.

ENVIRONMENT FACTS

- Here's a guide to how far the equivalent of a barrel of oil will take you in terms of energy.

  Walking – 16,000 km (London to Cape Town)
  Cycling – 53,900 km (one and a third times around the equator)
  Large car (3-litre diesel SUV) – 1,540 km (London to Lisbon, Portugal)
  Small car (1-litre engine) – 3,700 km (London to Newfoundland)
  Jumbo jet – 9 km (34 seconds of flying)

- Carbon footprint is such an overused term so, to clarify, it is the amount of greenhouses gases that your lifestyle produces, measured in tonnes. For example, two return flights to Mexico generate 4.9 tonnes of CO_2 emissions. The average carbon footprint for an individual is 10–12 tonnes per year. Google's carbon footprint is 1.5 million tonnes. You can offset your carbon footprint by doing something green, such as donating to a tree-planting charity. But be aware that consuming less and reducing carbon emissions is the ultimate aim.

- In 2013, we recycled 43.6 per cent of our waste – the target is 50 per cent by 2020, but there are worrying signs of the rate slowing down and even levelling off. Friends of the Earth argue that we could recycle or compost 80 per cent of our rubbish.

- 1 recycled tin can would save enough energy to power a TV for three hours.

- 1 recycled glass bottle saves enough to power a computer for 25 minutes.

- 1 recycled plastic bottle saves enough to fuel a 60-watt light bulb for three hours.

ACKNOWLEDGEMENTS

Thanks to Merope Mills, editor of the Saturday *Guardian*, who was so enthusiastic when I first came up with the 5:2 Your Life concept, and deputy editor Charlotte Northedge, who brought the idea to life brilliantly in *Weekend* magazine.

Thanks to my ever-encouraging agent Judith Murray and tireless editor Sarah Rigby, and the rest of the team at Hutchinson. Also to old friends Angela Hagan, Greta Sani, Stephen Johnstone, Clare Longrigg and Genevieve Fox for their advice and support. Thanks to Paul Heaney for suggesting 5:2 Your Productivity – I hope he finds it useful! And to Emily Cunningham for her excellent research skills.

Thanks to my family: my sister-in-law Christina Smyth who gave me some invaluable 5:2 insights along the way; my mother-in-law for letting me stay with her in Cornwall; my father who had every confidence that I'd cross the finishing line so quickly; and my mother who, as a psychotherapist, always inspired my interest in all things psychology.

Special thanks to my children, Louis, Evie and Amelia, for allowing me to 5:2 areas of their life almost always uncomplainingly; June Jones for being our family rock; and, above all, my husband Simon, for always being there. I look forward to his promised sequel – *5:2 Your Wife*!

I would also like to thank the many and numerous early adopters and testers who were willing to report back on what it's really like to 5:2 your life, and spread the word. I'm indebted, too, to the following experts for their ideas, inspiration and practical advice that have helped to shape this book. Their books and websites make for invaluable further reading.

Drink
Donna Cornett
Georgia Foster
Andrew Langford
Professor Chris Day
Jayne Totty
Catherine Salway

Fitness
Steve Mellor
Professor Maureen MacDonald
Chris Jordan
Professor John Brewer
Dr Costas Karageorghis

Finance
Merryn Somerset Webb
Simonne Gnessen
Professor Karen Pine

Productivity
David Allen
Richard Koch
Oliver Burkeman
Tony Schwarz
Graham Allcott
Fergus O'Connell

Screen
Dr Richard Graham
Professor Rose Luckin

Relationship
Professor John Gottman
Philippa Perry
Professor Janet Reibstein
Pamela Stephenson Connolly
Susanna Abse
Harriet Drake

Worry
Professor Mark Williams
Dr Robert Leahy
Dr Paul Jackson

Environment
Mike Berners-Lee
Joanna Yarrow
Julia Hailes

SELECTED BIBLIOGRAPHY

5:2 YOUR LIFE

Kidron, Beeban, 'We have abandoned our children to the internet', *Observer*, 13 September 2013

Day, Elizabeth, 'Hail the reviving power of summer', *Observer*, 31 August 2013

Duhigg, Charles, *The Power of Habit* (Random House, 2012)

Harvie, Michelle, and Tony Howell, *The 2-Day Diet* (Vermillion, 2013)

'5:2 Your Life', *Guardian Weekend* magazine, 15 June 2013

5:2 YOUR DRINK

Boniface, S., and N. Shelton, 'How is alcohol consumption affected if we account for under-reporting? A hypothetical scenario', *European Journal of Public Health*. first published online 26 February 2013: academia.edu/2703270/How_is_alcohol_consumption_affected_if_we_account_for_under-reporting_A_hypothetical_scenario

Cook, Emma, 'Is it six o'clock yet?', *Guardian*, 5 November 2005

Cornett, Donna, *Moderate Drinking Made Easy Workbook* (People Friendly Books, 2009)

Foster, Georgia, *The Drink Less Mind* book and hypnosis CD (Foster Publishing, 2006)

Holahan, Professor Charles, *et al.*, 'Late-life alcohol consumption and 20-year mortality', *Alcoholism: Clinical & Experimental Research*, 2010, 34(11), 1961–71: www.utexas.edu/news/2010/08/27/psychology_drinking/

Martínez-González, Miguel Ángel, *et al*, part of the *Predimed* report on the Mediterranean diet, 2013

Petri, A. L., *et al.*, Alcohol intake, type of beverage, and risk of cancer in pre- and postmenopausal women', *Alcoholism: Clinical & Experimental Research*, 2004, 28(7), 1084–90

Schütze, M., *et al.*, 'Alcohol attributable burden of incidence of cancer in eight European countries based on results from prospective cohort study', *British Medical Journal*, 2011, 342(d1584)

5:2 YOUR FITNESS

Bassett D., *et al.*, 'Pedometer-measured physical activity and health behaviors in U.S. adults', *Medicine & Science in Sports & Exercise*, 2010, 42(10), 1819–25

Bassett, D., *et al.*, 'Physical activity in an Old Order Amish community', *Medicine & Science in Sports & Exercise*, 2004, 36(1), 79–85

Gibala M. J., *et al.*, 'Physiological adaptations to low-volume, high-intensity interval training in health and disease', *The Journal of Physiology*, 2012, 590(5), 1077–84

Ingle, Sean, 'The Tabata workout programme: harder, faster, fitter, quicker?', *Guardian*, 25 March 2013

Karageorghis, C. I., *et al.*, 'On the role of lyrics in the music-exercise performance relationship', *Psychology of Sport and Exercise*, first published online 26 October 2013

Katzmarzyk, P. T., and I. Lee, 'Sedentary behaviour and life expectancy in the USA: a cause-deleted life table analysis', *BMJ Open*, 2012, 2(4)

Jordan, C. and Klika, B., 'High-intensity circuit training using body weight: maximum results with minimal investment', *Health & Fitness Journal*, 2013, 17(3), 8–13

Jordon, C. and Klika B., 'High-Intensity Circuit Training: The 7-Minute Workout', the Human Performance Institute, a division of Wellness & Prevention, Inc, a Johnson & Johnson Company

Levine, James, *Move a Little, Lose a Lot* (Crown Archetype, 2009)

Mellor, Steve, 'The four-minute 5:2 workout', head of personal training and nutrition, Freedom2Train

Murray, Jenni, 'Michael Mosley: "Three minutes of exercise a week will keep you fit"', *Radio Times*, February 2012

Pageaux B., S. M. Marcora and R. Lepers, 'Prolonged mental exertion does not alter neuromuscular function of the knee extensors', *Medicine & Science in Sports & Exercise*, first published online 21 May 2013

Reynolds, Gretchen, 'The rise of the minimalist workout', *New York Times*, 24 June 2013

Sim A.Y., K. E. Wallman, T. J. Fairchild and K. J. Guelfi, 'High-intensity intermittent exercise attenuates ad-libitum energy intake', *International Journal of Obesity*, first published online 4 June 2013

Tabata Dr I., K. Nishimura, M. Kouzaki, *et al.*, 'Effects of moderate-intensity endurance and high-intensity intermittent training on anaerobic capacity and VO2max', *Medicine & Science in Sports & Exercise*, 1996. 28(10), 1327–30

Trapp E. G., *et al.*, 'The effects of high-intensity intermittent exercise training on fat loss and fasting insulin levels of young women', *International Journal of Obesity*, 2008, 32(4), 684–91

5:2 YOUR FINANCE

Amis, Martin, *Experience* (Vintage, 2001)

Atalay, A. S., and M. G. Maloy, 'Retail therapy: a strategic effort to improve mood', *Psychology & Marketing*, 2011, 28(6), 638–59

Cryder, C., J. Lerner, J. Gross, and R. Dahl, 'Misery is not miserly: sad and self-focused individuals spend more', *Psychological Science*, 2008, 19(6), 525–30

Mani, A., *et al.*, 'Poverty impedes cognitive function', *Science*, 2013, 341 (6149), 976–80: www.sciencemag.org/content/341/6149/976

Pine, Karen, and Simonne Gnessen, *Sheconomics* (Headline, 2009)

Raghubir, P., and J. Srivastava, 'The denomination effect', *Journal of Consumer Research*, 2009, 36(4), 701–13

Somerset Webb, Merryn, *Love Is Not Enough: The Smart Woman's Guide to Money* (Harper Perennial, 2008)

5:2 YOUR PRODUCTIVITY

Allcott, Graham, *How to Be a Productivity Ninja* (Read Press, 2012)

Allen, David, *Getting Things Done* (Piatkus, 2002)

Ariga, A., and A. Lleras, 'Brief and rare mental "breaks" keep you focused: deactivation and reactivation of task goals preempt vigilance decrements', *Cognition*, 2011, 118 (3), 439–43

Burkeman, Oliver, *Help!: How to Become Slightly Happier and Get a Bit More Done* (Canongate, 2011)

Cirillo, Francesco, *The Pomodoro Technique* (Lulu.com, 2009)

Covey, Stephen R., *The 7 Habits of Highly Effective People* (Simon & Schuster, 2004)

Currey, Mason, *Daily Rituals* (Picador, 2013)

Ericsson, K. A., R. T. Krampe and C. Tesch-Römer, 'The role of deliberate practice in the acquisition of expert performance', *Psychological Review*. 1993, 100(3), 363–4006

Koch, Richard, *The 80/20 Manager: Ten Ways to Become a Great Leader* (Piatkus, 2013)

O'Connell, Fergus, *The Power of Doing Less* (Capstone, 2013)

Riedmann A., H. Bielenski, T. Szczurowska and A. Wagner, 'Working time and work–life balance in European companies', European Foundation for the Improvement of Living and Working Conditions, 2004–2005

Rosen, Michael and Helen Oxenbury, *We're Going on a Bear Hunt*, (Walker Books, 1997)

Tracy, Brian, *Eat That Frog* (Hodder, 2013)

Wieth, M. B., and R. T. Zacks, 'Time of day effects on problem solving: when the non-optimal is optimal', *Thinking & Reasoning*, 2011, 17(4), 387–401

5:2 YOUR SCREEN LIFE

Bavelier, Daphne, *et al.*, 'Improved probabilistic inference as a general learning mechanism with action video games', *Current Biology*, 2010, 23, 1573–9

Cook, Emma, 'Should we fear the iNanny?', *Guardian*, 27 April 2013

Cook, Emma, '5:2 your life – the screen diet', *Guardian*, 15 June 2013

'Children's and young people's reading today', National Literacy Trust, 2012: literacytrust.org.uk

Luckin, Rose, *Handbook of Design in Educational Technology* (Routlege, forthcoming)

Ofcom, 'The reinvention of the 1950s living room', 1 August 2013: http://media.ofcom.org.uk/2013/08/01/the-reinvention-of-the-1950s-living room-2/

Sigman, Aric, 'Time for a view on screen time', *Archives of Disease in Childhood*, 2012, 97(11), 935–42

Sullivan, Alice, and Matt Brown, 'Social inequalities in cognitive scores at age 16: The role of reading', CLS Working Paper Series, Institute of Education, 2013

Thomée, Sara, *et al.*, 'Computer use and stress, sleep disturbances, and symptoms of depression among young adults – a prospective cohort study', *BMC Psychiatry*, 2012, 12–176

Times Educational Supplement and E-Learning Foundation Survey 2010: http://www.bbc.co.uk/news/education-11738519

Wartella, Ellen, *et al.*, 'Parenting in the Age of Digital Technology', Center on Media and Human Development, School of Communication, Northwestern University, 2013

Wood, Clare, *et al.*, 'A longitudinal study of children's text messaging and literacy development', *British Journal of Psychology*, 2011, 102(3), 431–42

Ward, Victoria, 'Toddlers becoming so addicted to iPads they require therapy', *Daily Telagraph*, 21 April 2013

5:2 YOUR RELATIONSHIP

Charnetski C. J., and F. X. Brennan, 'Sexual frequency and salivary immunoglobulin A (IgA)', *Psychological Reports*, 2004, 94(3 Pt 1), 839–44

Gottman, John, and Nan Silver, *The Seven Principles for Making Marriage Work*, (Orion, 2007)

Grewen K. M., B. J. Anderson, S. S. Girdler, K. C. Light, 'Warm partner contact is related to lower cardiovascular reactivity',

Behavioral Medicine, 2003, 29(3), 123–30

Houlson, Catherine, *et al.*, 'Sleep, sex and sacrifice – the transition to parenthood, a testing time for relationships', OnePlusOne, 2013

Perry, Philippa, *How to Stay Sane* (Macmillan, 2012)

Reibstein, Janet, *The Best Kept Secret: How Love Can Last For Ever* (Bloomsbury, 2006)

5:2 YOUR WORRY

Bono, J. E., T. M. Glomb, W. Shen, E. Kim and A. Koch, 'Building positive resources: effects of positive events and positive reflection on work-stress and health' *Academy of Management Journal*, first published online 6 September 2012

Burkeman, Oliver, *The Antidote: Happiness for People Who Can't Stand Positive Thinking* (Canongate, 2013)

Cook, Emma, 'How to be happy in yourself', *Guardian*, 15 August 2005

Cohen, T., A. Panter and N. Turan, 'Guilt proneness and moral character, *Current Directions in Psychological Science*, 2012, 21(5), 355–9

Jackson, J., and E. Gray, 'Functional pear and public insecurities about crime', *British Journal of Criminology*, 2010, 50(1), 1–22

Kirby, Elizabeth D., *et al.*, 'Acute stress enhances adult rat hippocampal neurogenesis and activation of newborn neurons via secreted astrocytic FGF2', *Elife*, 16 April 2013

Leahy, Robert L., *The Worry Cure* (Piatkus, 2006)

Ramirez, Gerardo, and Sian L. Beilock, 'Writing about testing worries boosts exam performance in the classroom' *Science*, 2011, 331(6014), 211–13

Russ, T., *et al.*, 'Association between psychological distress and mortality: individual participant pooled analysis of 10 prospective cohort studies', *British Medical Journal*, 2012, 345(e4933)

Sample, Ian, 'Keeping a diary makes you happier', *Guardian*, 15 February 2009

Shiels, Chris, *et al.*, 'Evaluation of the statement of fitness for work (fit note): quantitative survey of fit notes', *Department for Work & Pensions*, 2013

Williams, Mark and Danny Penman, *Mindfulness: A Practical Guide to Finding Peace in a Frantic World* (Piatkus, 2011)

5:2 YOUR ENVIRONMENT

Berners-Lee, Mike, *How Bad Are Bananas?* (Profile Books, 2010)

Hailes, Julia, *The New Green Consumer Guide* (Simon & Schuster, 2007)

Howell, R. T., and G. Hill, 'The mediators of experiential purchases: determining the impact of psychological needs satisfaction and social comparison', *Journal of Positive Psychology.* 2009, 4(6), 511–22

Jaffrey, Madhur, *World Vegetarian* (Ebury, 1998)

Proud, Danielle, *House Proud: Hip Craft for the Modern Homemaker* (Bloomsbury, 2008)

Richins, M. L., 'When wanting is better than having: materialism, transformation expectations, and product-evoked emotions in the purchase process" (2013), *Journal of Consumer Research*, 2013, 40(1), 1–18

Yarrow, Joanna, *How to Reduce Your Carbon Footprint: 365 Practical Ways to Make a Real Difference* (Duncan Baird Publishing, 2008)

SELECTED
FURTHER READING

Berners-Lee, Mike, and Duncan Clark, *The Burning Question* (Profile Books, 2013)

Bittman, Mark, VB6: *Eat Vegan Before 6:00* (Sphere, 2013)

Dunn, Elizabeth and Michael Norton, *Happy Money: The New Science of Smarter Spending* (Oneworld Publications, 2013)

Harrison, Kate, *The 5:2 Diet Book.* (Orion, 2013)

Harvie, Michelle and Tony Howell, *The 2-Day Diet* (Ebury, 2013)

Heaversedge, Jonty and Ed Halliwell, *The Mindful Manifesto* (Hay House, 2012)

Mosley, Michael and Mimi Spencer, *The Fast Diet* (Short Books, 2013)

Northrup, Kate, *Money: A Love Story* (Hay House, 2013)

INDEX

Abel and Cole 250

Abse, Susanna 188

abstinence, periods of 9, 12, 13, 29, 157, 159

alcohol *see* drink, 5:2 your

Alcohol Research UK 31

Alcoholism: Clinical and Experimental Research 29

alcohol-free days (AFDs) 19, 31, 32, 34, 37, 42, 43, 45, 46, 50, 55, 56

Allcott, Graham 126, 130, 141, 143–4, 145, 146

Allen, David 128, 129, 142

American Institute for Cognitive Therapy, New York 215

Amis, Martin 92

Aniston, Jennifer 8

Antidote: Happiness for People Who Can't Stand Positive Thinking, The (Burkeman) 214

Apple 154, 155, 156

apps 84, 156, 166, 168, 176

Archives of Disease in Childhood 177

batch cooking 250–1

BBC 168

Berners-Lee, Mike 237, 238, 249, 250, 252, 252*n*, 254, 256, 257, 260, 263

Best-Kept Secret – How Love Can Last For ever, The (Reibstein) 182

Brailsford, Sir David 202

breast cancer 58, 233

breathing exercises 211, 216, 219–21, 224, 225–6, 228, 229–31

Brewer, Professor John 64

British Cycling 202

British Liver Trust 31, 35

Brunel University 83

Buddhism 13

buddy system 262–3

burpee 71–2, 74

Burke, Edmund 236

Burkeman, Oliver 128, 214

Capio Nightingale Hospital 158

carbohydrates 13, 14

carbon emissions/footprint:
    buying less and 256, 259
    carbon fuels, end of 241
    changing habits and 239
    diet and 248, 249, 252, 252*n*, 253, 254
    exercise and 265
    term 266
    textiles and 259
    transport and 17, 19, 236, 246, 260, 263, 264

Carnegie Mellon University, Pennsylvania 233

Centre for Alcohol Research, National Institute for Public Health, Denmark 58

Christianity 13

circuit exercises 63, 67, 69, 74–6, 79–81 *see also* fitness, 5:2 your

Cirillo, Francesco 149

climate change 238, 248, 249, 252*n*

Coco-politan 52

Cocorita 51–2

cognitive behavioural therapy (CBT) 213
Cornett, Diana 33, 36, 39, 45
cravings 13–14, 38, 44, 45, 48, 172, 214
credit crunch 234
Cycle to Work 112, 113
cycling 59
  children and 247
  environment and 21, 112, 113, 260, 261, 263, 265, 266
  goals and 165
  incidental activity and 81, 82
  intensity of 61, 63, 64, 67, 68, 80
  productivity and 151
  screen life and 169, 170,
  seven-minute workout and 76
  tabata and 61
  your relationship and 190, 191

Daily Rituals (Currey) 141
Day, Professor Chris 47
deadlines 10, 17, 139, 142
Department of Health 58
depression 57, 58, 177, 214, 234
digital detox 87, 120, 157, 158
Doing Something Different (DSD) 94, 175
Dowling, Tim 204–5
Drake, Harriet 202–3
drink, 5:2 your 11, 27–58, 87, 120–1, 232
  aims and benefits, 5:2 drink diet 31–2
  alcohol-free days (AFDs) 19, 31, 32, 34, 37, 42, 43, 45, 46, 50, 55, 56
  audit, do a drink 33–4
  be prepared 36–8
  breast cancer and 58
  children and 27, 28, 29, 33, 38, 40, 45, 46
  common questions 55–6
  don't forget the benefits 45–6
  drink facts 56–8
  5:2 your 27–58
  getting started on the 5:2 drink diet 32
  guidelines, government daily alcohol 35, 36, 57
  hypnotherapy and 42–3
  life before my 5:2 drink diet 27–30
  liver and 31, 32, 36, 46, 47–8, 57, 58
  making the 5:2 connection 30–1
  motivations, look at your 38–41
  red wine 45, 58
  savour your drink 48–54
  set goals 35–6
  seven steps to make the 5:2 drink diet work for you 33–54
  social drinking 30, 32, 33
  ten ways to slash your units, even on drink days 43–5
  what should I bear in mind for the other five days? 55
  which other 5:2 life areas combine well with my AFDs? 55–6
  which two days should I choose for my AFDs? 55
  why do I need to do this? 55
Drink Aware 47
'The Drink Less Mind' 37
Drink Link Moderation 33

e-Learning Foundation 178
Eat That Frog (Tracy) 140
Ecology Building Society 265
80/20 Principle, The (Koch) 140

Ellis, Albert 213
email:
    abstaining from 8
    addictive nature of 14, 154, 167
    capturing usage of 160, 161, 162, 163
    checking at home 18, 92
    children and 157
    clearing your inbox 128, 129–32, 134
    fast day and 164, 165
    5:2 143–4
    ignoring 135, 136
    relationship and 181, 186, 232
    screen life and 157, 160, 161, 162, 163, 164, 165, 167, 168, 172, 173, 174, 175
    telephone and 142
    weekends and 145, 147, 148, 151, 175
Energy Project 125, 148
environment, 5:2 your 21, 24, 87, 235–66
    aims and benefits, the 5:2 environment fix 239
    audit, do a green 240–3
    batch cooking 250–1
    be a 5:2 veggie 254–6
    be nice to yourself 262–3
    buddy system and 262–3
    buy less, spend less, buy better 256–8
    reject fast fashion 258–60
    carbon emissions/footprint 236, 238, 239, 241, 246, 248, 249, 252, 252n, 253, 254, 256, 259, 260, 264, 265, 266
    climate change 238, 248, 249, 252n
    common questions 265
    drink 253–4

energy 243–5
environment facts 266
flying 236, 263–4
food 249–52
getting started on the 5:2 environment fix 240
habits you can measure 243–7
life before my 5:2 environment fix 235–8
make it a joy not a duty 260–4
making the 5:2 connection 238–9
recycling 236–7, 266
seven steps to make the 5:2 environment fix works for you 240–64
'synergistic goals', aim for 260–2
take pleasure from 'beating the system' 262
think about how you eat 247–54
travel 245–7, 263–4
upcycle 259, 260
vegetarian diet and 238, 254–6
what other 5:2 life areas can I combine with the environment fix? 265
which two days should I choose to focus on the environment? 265
European Foundation for the Improvement of Living and Working Conditions 152
exercise see fitness, 5:2 your

Facebook 14, 131, 143, 145, 163, 173
FaceTime 155, 163, 164, 165, 176, 181
Fast Diet, The (Mosley) 62
fast days 10, 30, 35, 45, 55, 150, 164, 174, 176, 251
fasting 8, 10, 13, 30, 62, 93, 171, 204

Fearnley-Whittingstall, Hugh 255
finance, 5:2 your 11, 56, 87, 91–121, 175, 232, 265
  aims and benefits, 5:2 money diet 95
  audit, do a money 96–9
  common questions 120–1
  confront your money demons 109–11
  cut your fixed costs 106–9
  finance facts 121
  'frugality hackers' movement 112
  getting started on the 5:2 money diet 95
  life before my 5:2 money diet 91–3
  making the 5:2 connection 93–4
  money-free day (MFD) 102, 104, 111, 120
  restricted-money days (RMDs) 101–6, 112, 120
  Save It! App 112
  set goals 100–1
  seven steps to make the 5:2 money diet work for you 96–120
  seven ways to help cut your spending 111–14
  transport costs 112
  understand your money psyche 114–20
  which other 5:2 life areas combine well with my Money Diet? 120–1
  which two days should I choose? 120
  why do I need to do this? 120
fitness, 5:2 your 56, 59–89, 151, 174, 204, 265
  aims and benefits, 5:2 fitness plan 66–7

burpee 71–2, 74
circuit exercises 63, 67, 69, 74–6, 79–81
common questions 86–8
create the perfect playlist 84–6
cycling 21, 59, 61, 63, 64, 67, 68, 76, 80, 169, 170, 190, 191, 202, 236, 246, 260, 261, 263, 265, 266
feel the pain for a bit of gain 62–3
fitness facts 88–9
five ways to boast your incidental fitness 82–3
the four-minute 5:2 workout 71–4
the get-up 72
getting started on 67
goals 70
HIIT approach, is it right for you? 67–9 see also High-Intensity Interval Training (HIIT)
HIIT circuit, my first four-minute 74–6
HIIT flexibility, 5:2 79–81
hormesis 62
how will I feel when I do these exercises? 86
incidental activity 81–3
lean and mean 69–70
life before my 5:2 fitness plan 59–60
making the 5:2 connection 60–6
'the minimalist workout' 60
mix and match exercises 73–4
mountain climber and 72
music and 83–6
non-exercise activity thermogenesis (NEAT) 81, 89
plank push-up 73, 74
post-exercise high 69
post-exercise oxygen consumption (EPOC) 66, 88

running 20, 24, 59, 60, 63, 66, 67, 71, 72, 73, 76, 80, 81, 85, 86, 125, 148, 149, 164, 170, 260

set goals 69–71

seven steps to make the 5:2 fitness plan work for you 67–86

seven-minute workout, the ultimate 76–9

skipping rope 80

squat 72, 77, 79, 83

squat press 73, 74

swimming 63, 67, 80–1, 169, 170

tabata 61–2, 69, 71, 75, 79, 80, 82, 88, 125, 129, 147–50, 151

walking lunges 72, 74

what benefits can I expect to feel and see? 87

what days shall I do it on? 88

which other 5:3 life areas combine well with fitness? 87

5:2:

appreciation of food and 10, 32, 48–51

birth of 14–15

deprivation and 7, 22, 38, 118

first experience with 9–10

how long should I do it all for? 22–3

introducing to family 11, 12

it's fine to fail 23

making it work for you 20–2

'multi' approach 12

my journey on 20

psychological benefits 9–10

self-denial and 7, 91

spread of 8–9

success of 7

the philosophy 16–19

why these eight areas? 15

willpower and 7, 9, 10, 12, 17, 124, 125

Florida State University 152

flying 236, 239, 242, 253, 263–4, 266

Ford, Henry 14–15, 146

Foster, Georgia 37, 38, 39, 40, 42, 48, 49

43folders.com 129

Freedom2Train 63

Freud, Sigmund 212

Friends of the Earth 266

Getting Things Done (Allen) 128

Gibala, Martin 61

Gnessen, Simonne 102, 107, 110, 111–12, 119

Gottman, John 182, 194, 198, 199, 205, 206

Graham, Dr Richard 158, 160, 161, 162, 164, 166, 169, 170, 171, 172

Guardian 64

Guardian Weekend 12

Hailes, Julia 238–9, 244

heart disease 58, 59, 233

Help!: How to Become Slightly Happier and Get a Bit More Done (Burkeman) 128

High-Intensity Interval Training (HIIT) 87, 125–6

HIIT flexibility 79–82

is the HIIT approach right for me? 67–9

matching 5:2 with 63, 64, 65, 66

molecular changes and 88

my first four-minute HIIT circuit 74–6

screen life and 175

seven-minute workout 76–9

tabata and 61–2, 147–50
Hippocrates 13
Hopkinson, Simon 255
House Proud: Hip Craft for the Modern Homemaker (Proud) 259
How Bad Are Bananas? (Berners-Lee) 237, 263
How to Be a Productivity Ninja (Allcott) 126
How to Reduce Your Carbon Footprint: 365 Practical Ways to Make a Real Difference (Yarrow) 238
How to Stay Sane (Perry) 181–2
Howell, Ryan 258
Human Performance Institute, Florida 68, 76
hypnotherapy 37, 42–3

InRealLife (Kidron) 12
International Journal of Obesity 66
iPad 84, 153, 154, 156, 166, 167, 177, 204, 222
iPhone 12, 164
iPlayer 156
iPod 19, 153, 164
Islam 13

Jackson, Dr Paul 216, 222–3, 233
Jordan, Chris 67–8, 69, 76
Journal of Consumer Research 121

Karageorghis, Dr Costas 83–4
Kay, Steve 141
Klika, Brett 76

Langford, Andrew 31
laptops 12, 145, 146, 154, 155, 156, 158, 160, 164, 204, 257
Leahy, Robert L. 215, 216, 219, 223, 226, 227, 231

Lipman, Joanne 171
liver 31, 32, 36, 46, 47–8, 57, 58
Lleras, Alejandro 152
London School of Economic and Political Science 233
Luckin, Professor Rose 158, 160, 166, 168, 176

MacDonald, Professor Maureen 64, 65, 66, 68, 85
Mann, Merlin 129
marriage 182, 194, 198
Mauve Mary 54
MBCT (Mindfulness-Based Cognitive Therapy) 213, 214
McEwen, Simon 85
McMaster University, Ontario 61, 64
Meat Free Monday 255, 265
Medicine and Science in Sports and Exercise 89
meditation 19, 25
  alcohol and 41
  breathing exercises and 219–20
  fitness 68–9, 87
  productivity 130, 151
  screen life and 172
  your worry and 213, 214, 216–17, 219–20, 223, 225–6, 229, 230, 232
Mellor, Steve 63, 71, 74–5, 80, 81–2, 85, 86, 87, 88, 125
mental health 177, 234
Mindfulness: A Practical Guide to Finding Peace in a Frantic World (Penman/Williams) 18, 213
mindfulness meditation exercises 18–19, 41, 68–9, 87, 130, 151, 172, 213, 214, 216, 219–20, 223, 225–6, 229, 230, 232
Minecraft 158, 168

Mockito 53
money *see* finance
MoneyWeek 94
Mosley, Dr Michael 62, 81
mountain climber 72
Move a Little, Lose a Lot (Levine) 89
music 83–6, 152, 170–1

National Geographic 168
National Literary Trust 167
New Green Consumer Guide, The (Hailes) 238–9
New York Times 60, 170
NHS 13, 234
Nicholls, Dr James 31
non-exercise activity thermogenesis (NEAT) 81, 89
Northwestern University 161

O'Connell, Fergus 126, 132–3, 135–6, 139
Obama, Barack 63, 188
obesity 13–14, 48, 59, 66
Ofcom 177
OnePlusOne 206
'one-year-to-live' list 133–4
Oxfam 258
Oxford University 49, 213

Perry, Philippa 55, 181–2, 188, 192, 204
Pine, Professor Karen 94, 96, 102, 114, 175
plank push-up 72–3
Plato 13
Pomodoro technique 111, 129, 149, 150
post-exercise oxygen consumption (EPOC) 66, 88
Power of Doing Less, The (O'Connell) 126

Power of Habit, The (Duhigg) 18
pregnancy 9
procyanidins 58
productivity, 5:2 your 56, 87, 123–52
    aims and benefits, 5:2 productivity fix 127
    'bears' 140, 141
    common questions 151
    daily to-do list 134
    email and 129–32, 134, 135, 136, 142, 143–4, 145, 147, 148, 151 *see also* email
    getting started on the 5:2 productivity fix 127–8
    just say no 136–9
    life before my 5:2 productivity fix 123–5
    make your weekends sacred 145–7
    making the 5:2 connection 125–7
    most critical items 134–5
    'one-year-to-live' list 133–4
    Pomodoro technique 111, 129, 149, 150
    priority audit 132–6
    productivity facts 152
    'rocks' list 140, 141, 142
    set to zero 128–32
    seven steps to make the 5:2 productivity fix work for you 128–50
    slay your dragons 139–43
    'tabata' your workload 147–50
    thinking outside the box 131–2
    try 5:2 as a daily ratio 143–4
    what should I bear in mind for the other five days? 151
    which other 5:2 life areas combine well with productivity? 151

which two days should I choose to focus on 5:2 productivity? 151

working day, rhythm of 143–4

psychoanalysis/psychotherapy 212–14

Psychological Science 121

Psychology and Marketing 121

Q magazine 85

Race, Dr Phil 152

recycling 236–7, 240, 247, 252, 256–7, 259, 260, 266

Redemption 50

Reibstein, Professor Janet 182, 185, 186, 189–90, 191, 197, 198

relationship, 5:2 your 56, 118, 175, 179–207, 265

aims and benefits, the 5:2 relationship fix 183

audit, do a 'shared time' 184–7

babies and 206

build empathy 191–4

common questions 203–5

draw on the past 197–9

focus on the small things 202–3

four negative behaviours that are the doom of any relationship 'The Four Horsemen of the Apocalypse' 205

get to know each other 194–7

getting started on the 5:2 relationship fix 183–4

life before my 5:2 relationship fix 179–81

make a date 187–90

make a date with yourself 190–1

making the 5:2 connection 181–3

marriage 206

notes to self 196–7

relationship facts 205–7

seven steps to make the 5:2 relationship fix work for you 184–203

sex 200–1, 207

stress and 206–7

walk your way to a happy relationship 188–9

what should I bear in mind for the other five days? 204

which other 5:2 life areas combine well with relationships? 204–5

which two days should I choose to focus on my relationship? 203–4

Reynolds, Gretchen 60

Richins, Professor Marsha 258

Rose and Elderflower Cooler 53

Royal Marsden Hospital 233

running 24, 59, 72, 73

gratification of 60

high-intensity workout technique 20, 66, 67, 71, 80

playlist 85–6

productivity and 148

screen life and 164, 170

seven-minute workout and 76

time-consuming 60

Salway, Catherine 50

San Francisco State University 258

Schwarz, Tony 17, 125, 146, 147–9, 150

Screen Life, 5:2 your 12–13, 16, 87, 120, 147, 151, 153–78, 204, 232

aims and benefits, the 5:2 screen life diet; 158–9

audit, do a screen 159–63

be more mindful 171–3

common questions 173–6

computer games 178
digital dependency 154–5
do something different 170–1
family goals 166
getting started on the 5:2 screen
   life diet 159
house rules 164, 165
life before my 5:2 screen life diet
   153–4
make a plan 169
making the 5:2 connection
   157–8
'media-light'/'media-moderate'/
   'media-centric' families 161
mental disorders 177
screen life facts 177–8
set goals 165–7
set the rules 163–5
seven steps to make the 5:2
   screen life diet work for you
   159–73
sleep and 177, 222–3
something had to change 155–7
television 154, 156, 158, 160, 162,
   164, 169, 178
texting 160, 161, 163, 164, 167,
   168, 172, 173, 176, 178
think about quality, not just
   quantity 168–9
what changes can I expect after a
   few weeks on a 5:2 Screen Life
   Diet? 176–7
what should I bear in mind for the
   other five days? 174
which other 5:2 areas combine
   well with my Screen Life Diet?
   174–5
which two days should I choose
   for my Screen Life Diet?
   173–4
why do I need to do this? 173

7 Habits of Highly Effective People,
   The (Covey) 140
Seven Principles for Making Marriages
   Work, The (Gottman/Silver)
   182, 194, 198
sex 22, 183, 188, 195, 196, 200–1,
   206, 207
Sheconomics (Gnessen) 94, 102
shopping habits 11, 92
Sigman, Dr Aric 177
Silver, Nan 182, 194, 198
skipping rope 80
Skype 155
sleep:
   alcohol and 31, 222, 233
   exercise and 70, 87, 222, 233
   improvement in 11, 87, 222–3
   screen time and 177, 222–3,
      233
   worry and 211, 212, 215, 216,
      222–3, 233
squat 72, 77, 79, 83
squat press 73, 74
State of the Nation Report, The
   (2006) 206
Stephenson Connelly, Pamela 200,
   201
stress 21
   alcohol and 28, 39
   breathing exercises and 219–20
   finance and 116
   productivity and 149, 151
   screen life and 156, 177
   worry diet and 210, 215, 216,
      219–20, 233, 234
   your relationship and 195, 206
   see also worry 5:2 your
stroke 154, 233
Sullivan, Dr Alice 178
swimming 63, 67, 80–1, 169, 170

tabata 61–2, 69, 71, 75, 79, 80, 82, 88, 125, 129, 147–50, 151
Tabata, Professor Izumi 61, 147
Tavistock Centre for Couple Relationships 188, 202
Tavistock Clinic, London 158
Team Sky 202
television 82, 154, 156, 158, 160, 162, 164, 169, 178
Tesco 248–9
texting 14, 145, 160, 161, 163, 164, 167, 168, 172, 173, 176, 178, 181, 186
Think Productive 126
Thinking & Reasoning 152
Thomee, Sara 177
Times Educational Supplement 178
Timmons, Professor Jamie 62
Tokyo Iced Tea, A Simple 5:2 54
Totty, Jane 50, 51
travel 76, 106, 108, 133, 181, 236, 245–7, 260, 263–4
Twitter 14, 143, 145, 157, 173, 176

United Nations 248
University College London 33, 233
University of Bedfordshire 64
University of California 217, 219, 233
University of Coventry 178
University of Edinburgh 233
University of Gothenburg 177
University of Illinois 152
University of Kent 89
University of London 158, 178
University of Loughborough 62
University of Minnesota 219
University of Missouri 258
University of Newcastle 47, 57
University of North Carolina 206–7, 233

University of Rochester 178
University of Southern California 141
University of Texas 29
University of Western Australia 88
upcycle 259, 260

veg box, local 11, 250, 251, 253
vegetarian diet 238, 243, 254–6, 265
Vegetarian Research Group 255

walking lunges 72, 74
We're Going on a Bear Hunt (Rosen) 140
Webb, Merryn Somerset 94, 102, 104–5, 112, 113
weekends:
    alcohol and 28, 30, 35, 39, 40, 44, 49, 56
    exercise and 64, 85
    finance and 113, 120
    5:2 idea and 14–15
    indulgences during 24
    invention of 14–15
    make your weekends sacred 145–7
    productivity and 127, 128, 132, 145–7, 148, 151
    relationships and 8, 180, 188, 190, 191, 203
    screen life and 153, 154, 156, 159, 162, 167, 173, 175
weight loss 9, 11, 21, 45, 81
'When Wanting Is Better Than Having' (Richins) 258
Wilkes University, Pennsylvania 207
Williams, Professor Mark 18, 49, 50, 87, 172, 213–15, 216, 221, 225, 228, 229
Williams, Zoe 64

Wise Monkey Financial Coaching
    102
Wood, Professor Clare 178
worry, 5:2 your 87, 151, 209–34,
    265
  aims and benefits, the 5:2 worry
    diet 215
  audit, do a worry 217–19
  be kind to yourself 228–30
  breast cancer and 233
  breathing exercises 211, 216,
    219–21, 224, 225–6, 228,
    229–31
  cognitive behavioural therapy
    (CBT) 213
  common questions 231–2
  facts about worrying 233–4
  focus on the breath 219–21
  getting started on the 5:2 worry
    diet 215–16
  improve your sleep 222–3
  keep worry at bay on the other
    five days 230–1
  keep your worries in check 225–6
  keeping anxiety at bay 212–14
  life before my 5:2 worry diet
    209–10
  listen to what you are hearing and
    thinking 223–5
  make an appointment with your
    worries 227–8
  making the 5:2 connection
    214–15
  MBCT (Mindfulness-Based
    Cognitive Therapy) 213, 214

  mindfulness meditation/exercises
    18, 41, 130, 172, 213, 214, 216,
    219–20, 223, 225–6, 229, 230
  productive worry 226 7
  psychoanalysis/psychotherapy
    212–14
  rewind twenty years: my brush
    with anxiety 210–12
  seven steps to make the 5:2
    worry diet work for you 217–31
  sleep and 215, 216, 222–3
  sounds 223–4
  stress and 210, 215, 216, 219–20,
    233, 234
  tensing and relaxing 220, 221–2
  thoughts 225
  three-minute breathing exercise
    230–1
  tuning in to your thoughts 229
  what should I bear in mind for the
    other five days? 231–2
  which other 5:2 life areas
    combine well with my Worry
    Diet? 232–3
  which two days should I choose?
    231
  why do I need this? 231
  worry list 209, 218–19, 223, 226
Worry Cure, The (Leahy) 215

Yarrow, Joanna 238, 243, 245, 246,
    248, 250, 254, 255, 257, 258–9,
    262–3
YouTube 168